Reaching New Highs

Reaching New Highs
Alternative Therapies
For Drug Addicts

H. K. Heggenhougen, Ph.D.

JASON ARONSON INC.
Northvale, New Jersey
London

This book is based on an unpublished monograph, *Reaching New Highs: Turning "The Empty Fire"—Alternative Therapies for Drug Addiction*, prepared by H. K. Heggenhougen for Westover Consultants Inc., funded in part by the Substance Abuse and Mental Health Services Administration under Contract No. 277-91-1003. The author gratefully acknowledges permission to convert the monograph into this book.

Production Editor: Elaine Lindenblatt

This book was set in 11 pt. Cheltenham by Alpha Graphics of Pittsfield, New Hampshire and printed and bound by Book-mart Press of North Bergen, New Jersey.

Copyright © 1997 by Jason Aronson Inc.

10 9 8 7 6 5 4 3 2 1

All rights reserved. No part of this book may be used or reproduced in any manner whatsoever without written permission from Jason Aronson Inc. except in the case of brief quotations in reviews for inclusion in a magazine, newspaper, or broadcast.

Library of Congress Cataloging-in-Publication Data

Heggenhougen, Kris.
    Reaching new highs : alternative therapies for drug addicts / H. K. Heggenhougen.
        p. cm.
    Includes bibliographical references and index.
    ISBN 0-7657-0036-0 (alk. paper)
    1. Substance abuse—Alternative treatment.   2. Narcotic addicts—Rehabilitation.   3. Alcoholics—Rehabilitation.   I. Title.
RA564.H45   1997
616.86'06—dc20   96-35037

Printed in the United States of America on acid-free paper. For information and catalog write to Jason Aronson Inc., 230 Livingston Street, Northvale, New Jersey 07647-1731. Or visit our website: http://www.aronson.com

The lack of a calm inner tone in a person is described as a condition of "empty fire" (*xu huo*), because the heat of aggressiveness burns out of control when the calm inner tone is lost. It is easy to be confused by the *xu huo* that many addicts exhibit and to conclude that the main goal should be the sedation of excess fire. . . . [Rather] acupuncture helps patients with this condition to restore their inner control.

Smith and Khan 1988

Human beings are born with an innate need to get high, to experience periodically other states of consciousness, and the capacity for this experience is a capacity of the human nervous system.

External things may elicit highs, but the experiences are latent in our nervous systems, and their true causes are internal. It is possible to be high spontaneously and to learn to get high with less and less external stimulation.

Blum and Tilton 1981

Contents

Acknowledgments	ix
PART I **ALTERNATIVE THERAPIES FOR DRUG ADDICTS**	1
1 Introduction and Background	3
2 Traditional Medicine and Traditional Treatment of Addicts in Malaysia	15
3 Buddhist and Traditional Medical Therapies of Addicts in Thailand	35
4 Other Traditional and Herbal Therapies	41
5 Native American Therapies in the United States	47
6 Therapy through Alternative Achievements: Art Therapy and "Outward Bound" Revitalization	59
7 Biofeedback and Religious, Spiritual, and Meditation Therapies	67
8 Acupuncture Therapies	81
9 Salient Features of Alternative Therapies and Implications for Future Addiction Programs	87

PART II
ANNOTATED BIBLIOGRAPHY 93

1	Acupuncture	95
2	Affect/Psychology/Behavior	103
3	ASC/Hallucinogens/High Mind	105
4	Biofeedback/Relaxation	111
5	Various Countries/Thailand/Southeast Asia	113
6	Herbal Treatment	123
7	Ibogaine	125
8	Meditation/TM Treatment	129
9	Other	133
10	Psychodrama/Art Therapy/ Music Therapy/Books	139
11	Ritual/Spiritism/Revivalism/Spirituality in Treatment	141
12	Shamans	145
13	Therapeutic Communities/Outward Bound	149
14	Traditional Medicine	155

References   161

Supplemental Reading   187

Credits   201

Index   203

Acknowledgments

I should like to thank the many people who, in various ways, have helped in providing information and references for this study and in other ways have helped in its preparation and supported the author while he conducted this review. In particular I acknowledge the special skills of, and my appreciation of my friendship with, Abdul Rashid bin Abdul Razak, without whom the initial study carried out on alternative drug addiction therapies in Malaysia in 1978 and 1979 could not have been conducted; Myron Belfer and Arthur Kleinman for their encouragement; Anne Fitzgerald-Clark, Lisa Feldmann, and Melissa Cohen for their support and assistance in preparing the manuscript; the (library of the) Institute for the Study of Drug Dependence in London and its librarian for their hospitality and help in obtaining much of the relevant literature; Dr. Vichai Poshyachinda in Thailand, Dr. Hans Christian Sorhaug in Norway, and Dr. Margaret Patterson in the United States, to mention but three of the people who provided special references and took the time to discuss this project; Elaine Lindenblatt for her editorial help; and finally Maria Christina Ritz for her support and encouragement, in the face of the sun and sea.

PART I
Alternate Therapies for Drug Addicts

1
Introduction and Background

The misuse of drugs is a worldwide problem of drastic proportions and has appropriately received much publicity. Figures indicate that in most countries the number of drug-dependent addicts has increased over the last decade. The problem is particularly acute in Southeast Asia, a region including the "Golden Triangle," which supplies a considerable proportion of the world's opium—and thus heroin. In Malaysia, for example, the use of heroin (the most prevalent addictive drug) doubled between 1975 and 1980 when some estimates indicated there were more than 300,000 addicts in the Peninsular Malaysian population of 14 million people. Since then drug addiction has increasingly received national attention as a major social problem needing urgent action. But it is clear that the use and abuse of addictive drugs and alcohol are not limited to a particular region or to a small group of countries—it is perniciously pervasive throughout the world.

The cultural, social, political, and economic causes and consequences of this problem have been discussed at length elsewhere and will not receive major attention here. What should be noted, however, is that the treatment and rehabilitation programs that are most successful not only address the detoxification and the physical aspects of addiction but also incorporate in the treatment/rehabilitation program an understanding of the wide range of causative factors as well as the cultural and socioeconomic context of the addict. Thus, means of empowering the addict, especially in terms of re-creating a strong identity and positive self-image, as well as providing coping skills for dealing with the real world, are seen by these programs as crucial. Within a public health perspective, rather than the treatment of individual addicts, however, it is crucial not only to critically analyze, and be guided by an understanding of, the broad range of causative factors, which can never be limited to a matter of "personality deficiencies" and individual psychopathology, but also to consider how changes can be effected upon wider sociocultural, economic, and political circumstances.

These are the so-called pull factors that influence demand, and it is my conviction that demand reduction is ultimately far more important than supply reduction. Yet, possibly because the "enemy" can be more easily identified, it is supply reduction that has received a disproportionate amount of attention and resources from the "wars on drugs" mounted by most governments. But unless governments and others involved at policy levels are willing to engage in the more politically difficult task of examining and addressing socioeconomic characteristics linked with high rates of addiction (even if not seen as direct causes of addiction), new supplies are bound to replace those that have been stopped. As we review alternative therapies used throughout the world and consider their effectiveness and possible adaptability for therapeutic interventions in other settings, including the United States, we must recognize that such therapies may be extremely effective in healing and rehabilitating individual addicts but will probably only minimally affect the prevalence of drug addiction as such. For that, a much larger public health perspective must be employed that involves shifting the therapeutic focus from the individual to the community and society. But the elements deemed important in many alternative therapies of individual addicts may also guide such a wider purview.

Vast sums are spent by the United States and other countries on preventing the flow of drugs and on treatment and rehabilitation programs. Despite these national and international efforts the drug tide remains undiminished and no treatment/rehabilitation program can claim particular success. In the last several years, since the experiments of Wen (Wen and Cheung 1973) in Hong Kong, attention has focused on the use of acupuncture in drug dependence treatment and interest is increasing in other traditional, or alternative, and folk methods of treating addicts.

While recognizing that no one therapeutic program can be consistently the best or most appropriate for all addicts across national boundaries—individual, cultural, and other characteristics will influence the appropriateness of specific programs for individual patients from particular sociocultural contexts—the almost uniform lack of success of standard, hospital-based addiction therapy programs makes us turn to the mounting evidence and promising reports of the efficacy of alternative therapies being used to rehabilitate addicts in different parts of the world, including North America and Europe. But it is not only the appallingly poor performance of the orthodox programs that would interest us in other approaches; many of the alternative programs contain therapeutic elements that seem to contribute to their apparent success, even if only for specific groups of addicts. A few efficacy follow-up studies of alternative programs indicate a success rate far superior to that of orthodox methods; these warrant further studies.

In addition to reviewing some of these approaches, which is the main purpose of this book, it is also important both to note how these alternative programs differ from standard hospital-based programs, and to determine whether these programs have certain basic, universal characteristics which, if adapted to the circumstances of addicts on the spectrum of specific sociocultural and economic contexts, could improve addiction therapies in general. What are some of these alternative therapies? What do they do, and whom do they treat? What can we learn from them?

History of Opiate Use/Abuse

The use of psychotropic substances is not new; some say it goes back at least 20,000 years (LaBarre 1972). It appears to have been particularly widespread in Central America, where, for example, the culture of pre-Columbian Mexico has been described as "narcotic-oriented" (Schultes 1977). Furst (1972) and Harner (1973) provide further documentation of the widespread and longtime use of psychotropic drugs in South, Central, and North America. Hamarneh (1972) states that the use and misuse of drugs was widespread in urban, wealthy, and progressive centers of Arabia. The use of opium, khat, and hemp/hashish is not a recent phenomenon but has been described as having been prevalent in Asia Minor, North Africa, Persia (Iran), and India for at least a thousand years and most probably considerably longer. The first-hand description of drug use in seventeenth-century Asia by the German physician Kaepfer is but one of many interesting accounts (Bowers and Carrubba 1978). The current practice of coca leaf chewing by Quechua and Aymara Indians in Peru has its origins in the Inca past (Martin 1970, Negrete 1978, Petersen 1977). A number of examples have been documented at length by LaBarre (1975, 1977).

Some have argued, however, that the drug abuse and dependence we see today has had a relatively short history. In Asia it has been tied to the commercial interests of colonial powers in India and in Southeast Asia, resulting in the opium wars, in which opium was forcibly introduced into China against its will in order to stimulate commerce for the East India Company (Lowinger 1977, McCoy 1972). In a more general way it is also seen as one of the detrimental consequences of the breakdown of traditional cultures attributed by some to Western influences. It is an oversimplification of complex etiological phenomena, and debatable historically, to attribute the current addiction epidemic solely to the spread of Western civilization and thus to consider it a Western disease. But it is important to note that this connection is often made and it may offer a valid point of view (one of many) of the problem. It may also foster interest in, and the possible success of, alternative therapies, such as those of traditional and folk practitioners, in treating and rehabilitating addicts.

Although the literature is not lacking in documenting the pervasiveness and substantial history of drug abuse, until the 1970s it was sparse indeed concerning traditional and other alternative therapies or management of drug dependence. One explanation may be that despite the probable existence of addiction in various parts of the world, and at different periods, the great majority of drug taking was not associated with addiction and was integral to magico-religious ceremonies and healing rituals, reserved for special occasions, and often limited in scope. It was usually not taken at the frequency or in the secular manner of most contemporary drug (ab)use, which is not to say, as Agar (1973, 1975) has pointed out, that most present-day use is devoid of ritual. In other circumstances drug use might have been so pervasive (but not socially dysfunctional and thus not socially disruptive) that no sanction was issued against it and no pressure was put on individuals to cease their addiction maintenance. One may further question, for example, whether the opium-using hill tribes of Thailand or the coca-chewing Inca descendants in Peru who still use drugs, largely for medicinal reasons and to endure strenuous working conditions, can be classified as drug abusers, belonging to the same category as urban junkies.

The causes of addiction are many and multifactorial, but there is good cause to link at least a substantial proportion of the problem to rapid social change and to social, economic, and cultural (and ethnic) marginalization of individuals and groups—the making of the "other"—including diminishing respect for them and thus dismissing their dignity. Although this covers a great deal of ground it is an oversimplification of a far more complex etiology, which also differs in groups within and across countries. Yet I believe this perspective is sufficiently valid to offer at least a starting point from which to examine the problem and to interpret the relative success of alternative therapeutic practices.

In addition to noting the evidence concerning the pharmacological and biological efficacy of a number of herbal detoxification remedies, and the detoxification ability of acupuncture, the probable reason for the comparatively more favorable results of alternative therapies is the attention given to the wider socioeconomic and cultural factors contributing to or associated with drug abuse. The restoration of dignity and a positive identity as well as provision of means of coping in the everyday world are often central elements of alternative rehabilitation programs. For some, this has meant the rejuvenation of so-called traditional, including religious, values, or the adaptation of healing mechanisms previously used by particular ethnic groups (e.g., Native Americans). The symbolism of the "empty fire" (Smith and Khan 1988) is also relevant not only to the rehabilitative use of acupuncture but also to many alternative therapies that can be seen not as extinguishing the fire within but as enabling the former addict both to control his internal fire and, by means other than the use of exogenous drugs, to change the emptiness into a creative force with the potential for euphoria.

Traditional Medicine and Addiction Treatment: General Overview

The decade of the 1970s saw a resurgence of interest in traditional medicine that is still gathering strength. This was influenced by visits of international health personnel to China, whose reports focused worldwide attention on the use of traditional Chinese medicine including acupuncture (Chen 1972, Quinn 1972, 1974, Sidel and Sidel 1973, 1974). The World Health Organization has legitimized this concern and has passed several resolutions calling on member nations to incorporate traditional medicine into the official health care programs wherever and whenever possible (WHO 1975, 1976, 1977). In 1978 the Alma Ata Conference on Primary Health Care, emphasizing "health for all by the year 2000" (which would include rehabilitation from addiction), again suggested that consideration be given to the incorporation of traditional healers into national health care systems (WHO/UNICEF 1978). Many nations have taken steps toward such integration and the number of institutes for the study of traditional medicine is increasing. Traditional healers are generally thought of in terms of primary health care for rural populations, but they are also prominent in urban settings and their potential for the treatment of drug addiction has been expressed and is currently in practice in a number of settings.

Traditional medical practices of various kinds, belonging to both regional and local (or folk) systems (Dunn 1976) as well as syncretic or amalgam practices, are known to be used in the treatment of drug addiction (and alcoholism) in many countries. Such practices also include religious revivalism, faith healing, and rejuvenation rituals, as well as acupuncture, biofeedback, hypnosis, yoga, and different forms of meditation (Baer 1981, Benson 1969, Bourne 1975, Clements et al. 1988, Denney et al. 1991, Jilek 1989, 1993, Nelson 1975, Prince 1988, Ripinsky-Naxon 1989, Schuster 1975, Valla and Prince 1989). It is worth noting that much of traditional/alternative practice is not as dichotomized as cosmopolitan medicine and often relates to the total body-mind-spirit complex (Morinis 1978). Aspects of traditional healing practices, which from a Western scientific point of view seem unrelated to healing, are seen as such by these approaches and can be particularly effective with both the physical and psychosocial aspects of the problem of addiction.

Religion and drug/alcohol addiction rehabilitation have been linked for a long time. Many cured addicts become very religious. Drug taking itself has become a religion for some people and, conversely, there is probably much truth to the belief that religion is a positive opiate substitute. ("Religion is the opiate of the masses!"?) A number of studies point to the connection between religion and rehabilitation of drug addicts and claim that the intensity of religious involvement relates directly to the reduction of drug addiction and to the maintenance of abstinence (Beer 1981, Buxton et al. 1987, Galanter and Buckley 1978, Galanter et al. 1979, Singer 1982, Smith 1994, Westermeyer and Walzer 1975, Wilson 1972). A range of religious groups, from the orthodox to the esoteric, including faith healers, seem to be involved in the effort to rehabilitate addicts. In Mexico, for example, "espiritistas" are known to be working with drug addicts (Richards 1979). In the United States studies of the peyote rituals conducted by the Native American Church indicate their apparent positive effect on drug addicts and alcoholics, presumably due to both the religious aspects and the pharmacological properties of the peyote (Blum et al. 1977, Hill 1990) (see Chapters 3, 5, and 7).

Meditation, especially the practice of transcendental meditation, has also attracted recent attention and a number of studies point to a positive correlation between such practices and the reduction of drug-taking behavior (Anderson 1977, Benson and Wallace 1972, Clements et al. 1988, Gelderloos et al. 1991, Schuster 1975, Shaffi et al. 1975, Suwaki 1979). Other studies have shown that meditative practices can cause physiological changes, and it is possible that such changes inhibit a craving for addictive drugs (Pelletier 1977, Wallace 1970, Wallace and Benson 1972). It is conceivable, as some researchers have postulated, that such physiological changes could affect endorphins by influencing biochemical changes, such as the concentration of sodium in the cerebrospinal fluid, which in turn influence the opiate receptors (Blum and Tilton 1981, Lex and Meyer 1977, Lex and Schor 1977, Marx 1975, Patterson et al. 1993, Prince 1988, Snyder et al. 1974, Valla and Prince 1989).

A provocative article, "A Proposed Bioanthropological Approach Linking Ritual and Opiate Addiction," by Lex and Schor (1977), opened avenues for further investigation of traditional means of treating addicts. Lex and Schor proposed that there are neurobiological relationships among seemingly disparate phenomena—religious ritual, native curing therapies, and pharmacodynamic, psychological, and sociocultural components of drug addiction.

> It appears plausible that certain preparations for rituals—among them sweatbaths, fasting, emesis, and purgation—effectively decrease the amount of sodium in cerebrospi-

nal fluid below the normal level. In this manner the intracerebral environment is more conducive to activation of the opiate receptors by the endogenous morphine-like substance. [p. 295]

Jilek (1978, 1989, 1992, 1993a,b), Prince (1988), and Valla and Prince (1989) are some of the others who have discussed this interrelationship in more recent articles.

One may question whether alternative therapeutic methods, as they occur in Malaysia, Thailand, or elsewhere, affect the opiate receptors and possibly create a sense of well-being, if not euphoria, which minimizes the loss of the heroin (exogenously) produced "high." It should not be overlooked that causes for addiction and elements favoring successful rehabilitation of addicts are multifactorial and the questions generated by Lex and Schor are therefore particularly pertinent as they arise from both sociocultural and neurobiological considerations. Once again, a more integrated therapeutic approach is called for than is usual for most orthodox programs.

Until recently the literature describing the studies and experiences of alternative therapeutic approaches in treating and rehabilitating addicts focused on the use of acupuncture. The use of acupuncture for the treatment of addiction was discovered accidentally by Dr. Wen in Hong Kong in 1972 (Wen and Cheung 1973, Kao and Lu 1974). This use has now spread to other parts of the world, including Southeast Asia, Australia, Europe, and the United States (Lau 1976, Sainsbury 1974). Patterson (1974, 1977), who worked with Wen in Hong Kong, established an acupuncture addiction treatment center in England and claimed success with the method. She is particularly convinced about the efficacy of electrostimulation (Patterson 1993). She has reported on the invention of a portable stimulator that the patient could use whenever feeling a drug craving, thus obviating dependence on a special practitioner or treatment center.

It is still not known exactly how acupuncture works but experiments have shown that the stimulation from acupuncture needles produces an increased amount of endogenous opiate-like chemicals (Schmeck 1977) that might be significant in the reduction of withdrawal symptoms and drug craving. Most of the reports on acupuncture treatment of drug addicts are optimistic about the achievements of this method and about the potential for the future. While it is fairly well established that acupuncture is effective in providing significant relief to patients during detoxification, it is less certain whether it contributes to greater long-term abstinence rates. A few reports are careful to distinguish between treatment and rehabilitation and to make disclaimers about the tenacity of abstinence through the use of this method (Kao and Lu 1974).

Whitehead's (1978) review of studies responsible for the high regard given to acupuncture addiction treatment challenged the adequacy of clinical trials and the limited patient follow-up of early studies. One wonders, for example, how Severson and colleagues (1977), in a study published in the *International Journal of the Addictions* but not discussed by Whitehead, could speak of comparable relapse rates when discussing only eight patients, most of whom returned to drug use. More recently Riet and colleagues (1990) also conducted such a review with mixed results. Evaluation of acupuncture programs is still not substantial enough to warrant a definitive statement on the method (see Chapter 8).

In addition to acupuncture, other alternative methods are used in different parts of the world to treat addicts; for example, in Asia reports of the efforts of Hakkims come from Pakistan, of folk healers from Myanmar (U Khant 1985), of priests and folk healers from Thailand and Laos, and of bomohs (folk healers) treating addicts in Malaysia. There are religious Sheiks who treat addicts in at least 10 percent of Cairo's mosques in Egypt (Baasher and Abn el Azayem 1980), various traditional methods are used to treat alcoholism in Japan (Suwaki 1980), and in Alaska and in other circumpolar regions methods similar to those of Native American therapies in the United States are used (Mala 1985). There is Buddhist treatment of alcoholism in Sri Lanka (deSilva 1983), and yoga and other traditional approaches are used to treat several thousand addicts at the Nav-Chetna Center in India (Sharma and Shukla 1988). And the list goes on.

There is now a growing literature describing and evaluating the efficacy of these approaches. This book reviews this material and provides an annotated bibliography of some of the most prominent and/or interesting studies in this literature. Many of these approaches are effective, and an examination of them will provide important lessons for how to redesign so-called orthodox addict therapeutic programs and preventive efforts.

2

Traditional Medicine and Traditional Treatment of Addicts in Malaysia

In Malaysia, where the problem of addiction has seriously increased since 1975, a number of heroin addicts have turned to traditional folk healers (bomohs) for treatment. Heroin addiction is a recent phenomenon in Malaysia, but traditional Malaysian therapies for other forms of addiction have existed for a long time. Gimlette and Thomson (1939) mention the use of the biak leaf (*Mitragyne speciosa*), which was chewed as an opium substitute by addicts in Perak State to overcome their addiction; the practice apparently came from Thailand, where it had existed for some time (Burkill and Haniff 1930). Both Emboden (1972) and LaBarre (1975) refer to its use as an opium substitute under the names of *Kratom* and *Mambog* in Thailand and Singapore. In Telok Anson, Perak State, the biak leaves were made into a tea that was drunk by opium addicts.

Malaysia has one of the best national, cosmopolitan (allopathic) health center systems in the Southeast Asian region. Less than 10 percent of the rural population lives more than three miles from a government health center. Heavy reliance is placed on the services provided by this system, in both urban and rural areas. But, as in most countries, traditional systems of medicine are used as well. Traditional Chinese, Indian Ayurvedic, Siddha, and homeopathic and Malaysian folk (bomoh) health care resources are used for physical and psychological ailments either instead of the official system or in addition to it. The health care system in Malaysia is one of medical pluralism (Heggenhougen 1980a,b), with the traditional systems corresponding to the major ethnic groups in the country, although members of one ethnic group sometimes also use the traditional health care resources of another ethnic group. Despite the multiplicity of use by patients of resources belonging to various health care systems, there is relatively little contact or cooperation among these systems.

The first conference to bring together practitioners of traditional medicine and especially those concerned with drug addiction therapy was held at the University of Malaya in May 1979, with more than 300 representatives from the different traditional systems. Subsequently the Federation of the Malaysian Associations of Traditional Medicine was formed. Both of these efforts were initiated by the leadership of the Malaysian Association of Traditional Malay Medicine, which also was carrying out a special campaign to gain recognition for the bomohs who treated addicts, for example by promoting media coverage of the work of a few of the drug bomohs. Many in the association felt that Western/scientific methods had failed both to check the spread of addiction and to treat and rehabilitate addicts, and thus one should now turn to methods that are particularly Malaysian, founded on the country's traditions. The implication of this was that traditional medicine should be considered as neither stagnant nor backward but, according to Dunn (1975), "although firmly rooted in tradition it is also a modern, innovative, changing system" (p. 298). Traditional medicine was proposed as particularly relevant to the treatment of drug addiction, as cultural/psychological/social stress, loss of self-esteem, and an increased identity crisis have been mentioned as causes of addiction.

Chinese Traditional Medicine

In Peninsular Malaysia there are more than 1000 Sinsehs (traditional Chinese physicians) and a similar number of Chinese herbal shops. Kuala Lumpur has a training institute that has graduated several hundred Sinsehs who have attended a four-year course. Most Sinsehs belong to the Chinese Physicians Association. There are traditional Chinese hospitals in both Kuala Lumpur and Penang, and astrologers, palmists, temple mediums, and special temple prayers are resources also used by those seeking a solution to their ailments or problems (Chen 1981, Dunn 1974, 1975).

Apart from acupuncture (see Chapter 8), there are a few other traditional Chinese means of treating addicts. Many Chinese medicine shops sell a relatively inexpensive liquid made in Hong Kong known simply as the "Four-day-breaking-smoking-habit-medical-solution," which brings about vomiting when it is ingested and is reputed to be able to cure opium and heroin addiction when taken in larger doses and for a longer period than when used to stop cigarette smoking. According to the Sinseh in one Chinese medicinal shop, dried poppy shells are included in another mixture with "other ingredients" generally used to "strengthen the body" but which can also be taken as a tea by an opium/heroin addict withdrawing from drugs.

Early references reported the use of an "anti-opium leaf" (*Combretium sundaicum*), which was supposedly used by Chinese opium smokers in various parts of Southeast Asia who wanted to stop their habit (Hare et al. 1909, McBride 1910). Inquiries made at a number of medicinal shops in Kuala Lumpur, Ipoh, and Penang, however, were not able to confirm the current use of this plant.

It is reputed that one of the Chinese secret societies is treating heroin addicts in Penang, but this is hardly connected to traditional medicine as their method is apparently similar to that of Synanon.

Traditional Malay Medicine

It was estimated that there were 20,000 part-time folk healers (bomohs) in Malaysia in 1970 (Chen 1975), which, with an approximate population of 13 million people, meant a ratio of one bomoh for every 650 people. There is little indication that this ratio has decreased within the last 20 years. Some of these healers are now treating heroin addicts.

Although bomohs have a number of common characteristics, there are many differences among them. There is little standardization of training because even though some old texts are used (usually of Javanese and Arab origin), most bomohs become healers by learning from their bomoh father, from a special teacher (guru), or by receiving knowledge through a dream in which a special spiritual/supernatural encounter is experienced. Bomohs are also said to gain power by becoming the possessors of special helping spirits, such as a *hantu raya*, a *pelisit*, or a *polong* (Chen 1975, Heggenhougen 1980b, Mohd. Taib Osman 1972, 1976).

The folk healers may be classified as herbalists, spiritualists, or bone setters, or a combination of them. Those bomohs who know and use herbal cures also use special supernatural as well as Koranic *jampi-jampi* (incantations) when treating patients. Mohd. Taib Osman (1976) has called the bomoh a combination of "shaman, herbalist, diviner, curer and psychiatrist" (p. 26). There are bomoh generalists, but usually a bomoh is known for his (or her) ability to treat a set of specific ailments.

Much has been written about traditional bomoh medicine (Burkill and Haniff 1930, Chen 1970a,b, 1973, 1975, Colson 1971, Gimlette 1915, Gimlette and Burkill 1930, Heggenhougen 1980a,b,

McKay 1971, Mohd. Taib Osman 1972, 1976, Ridley 1906, Skeat 1900, Wolff 1965), but there is no standard description giving an overview of current practices and practitioners. The Association of Traditional Malay Medicine, which was established in May 1979, is unable to provide much information characterizing the practice of its membership. Similarly, the Association of Traditional Malay Medicine Sellers, initiated in 1974, cannot easily provide a descriptive overview of their members nor of the medicines involved (Heggenhougen 1980b). The Malaysian National Museum has a Division on Traditional Medicine with the purpose of collecting information on traditional bomoh medicine and on the medical practices of the Orang Asli (aboriginal people); it is hoped that the work of this group will be able to provide an overall documentation of such ongoing traditional practices.

Based on the various published accounts and interviews with different people concerned with drug addiction in Malaysia, I estimated that a minimum of at least a thousand heroin addicts had received treatment from bomohs by 1980. As the practice has continued, the number is considerably larger today. Drug bomohs do not treat their patients alike, but certain similarities can be seen. All of the healers use one or more medicinal vegetal concoctions during the detoxification/withdrawal phase. Such concoctions are given regularly for only three days by one bomoh and for a month or more by others; a few provide such concoctions for consumption subsequent to withdrawal and after the period of direct treatment/rehabilitation from the bomoh, to be taken whenever the patient craves drugs. The treatment usually lasts two to four weeks, during which time most of the bomohs have the patients live with them in the bomohs' homes.

All bomohs are Muslim and their treatment procedures include a spiritual component. Koranic incantations are used, the patients are encouraged to pray regularly, and Islamic religious sessions are held, which include repeated, rhythmic oral readings from the Koran. Some bomohs will perform special *pembenci* (hatred) charms and give special cleansing baths and massages. One bomoh even writes Koranic verses in Jawi script on the bodies of his patients. Some patients have claimed that they will not return to drug use because they fear that the bomoh's familiar spirit, his *hantu raya*, will make their lives miserable should they do so. It has been assumed that most bomohs are secretive and unwilling to cooperate with anyone interested in them, but during studies carried out by the author in the 1970s this was found to be untrue. The bomohs are not reticent; they freely discuss the manner of their treatments. This openness has also been reported by others. As is the case in general with practitioners the world over, however, some initial reluctance exists in revealing the exact recipe of their medicinal concoctions. At first they will talk in generalities and state only that their medicine contains "four kinds of roots and four kinds of herbs," or "five or six kinds of leaves, five or six kinds of roots, and a few tubers." But when the seriousness of the inquiry is established they tend to be more specific. The ingredients are gathered by the bomohs themselves and/or are bought from medicine root sellers and distributors in Malaysia, Singapore, and Indonesia. Some of the ingredients are bought from the Chinese medicinal shops and from Indian spice sellers.

The concoctions vary from the simple to the complex. One bomoh uses simply a combination of water, sugar, and *asam jawa* (sour fruit or tamarind—*Tamarindus indica*); another has his patients sit in a room smelling the *buah mengkudu* (fruit of the *Morinda elliptical Linne*); a third claimed that *daun Ketam*, also known as *daun gaudarusa* (leaves of *Geudarussa vulgaris*) was effective in "curing" addicts, while other medicines contain, according to one of the bomohs, up to "forty-four herbal, root, wood, fruit and leaf items." Some bomohs accuse each other of including opium as one of the ingredients in their medicines, but two samples we obtained from bomohs during our 1979 study in northwestern Malaysia (Perlis) were analyzed by the Department of Pharmacy of the Universiti Sains Malaysia and found to contain no opiates. Both samples did contain cinchona and indole alkaloid, however, and one sample contained cannabidiol and cannabinol.

One bomoh, being initially more open about his ingredients, stated that one of the concoctions he uses is a ground mixture of *daun pegaga* (the leaf of the creeping herb—*Hydrocotyle asiatica*) and *daun kunyit* (turmeric leaf—*Curcuma domestica*) mixed in water. The *daun pegaga* is widely used in traditional Malaysian folk medicine for the treatment of cough, vertigo, consumption, asthma, and disorders of the liver, and *daun kunyit* is used traditionally as an antispasmodic and carminative (Gimlette and Thomsen 1939).

The same bomoh also named all of the twenty-three ingredients of another concoction that his patients take internally in small amounts and use externally as an ointment during massage. It contains a number of turmeric and ginger roots (*Curcuma domestica*; *Zingiber ottensii*; *Z. officionale*; *Z. cassumunar*; *Kaempferia galanga*; and a rhizome of the genus *Languas-Koenig*), leaves of the white hibiscus (*Hibiscus rosasinensis*), root of the grass *Imperata cylindrica* (*akar lalang*), wood of the dragon shrub (*Mesua ferrea*), sweet flag (*Acorus calamas*), leaves and root of the *Allomorphis alata* (*puding hitam*), citronella grass (*Cymbopogon nardus*), leaves and roots of the *Hydrococtyle asiatica* (*pegaga*), roots of the "stone banana" and *daun pemalut burung bubut* (probably the leaves of the *Clerodendron villosum*), and *daun balik angin* (probably the leaves of the *Mallotus macrostachyus*). These ingredients are well powderized, mixed with *minyah kelapa hijan* (*santan*) (oil from the pulp of a green coconut), and given as a drink to the patients (translation of

Malay terms used by the bomoh to botanical names are from Burkill 1966, Burkill and Haniff 1930, Gimlette and Thomsen 1939).

Many of the ingredients mentioned are used by other bomohs to treat such different ailments as headache, flatulence, blood poisoning, asthma, jaundice, and malaria. Some allegedly are aphrodisiacs. Gimlette and Thomson (1939) pointed out that *Jerangau*, the Malay term for sweet flag, was used in Europe to cure the tobacco chewing habit and, in combination with other ingredients, it has been ingested by people in Malaysia to combat malaria and rheumatism. The *puding hitam* leaves are used to obtain good appetite, the *serai* grasses (*cymbopogon*) are supposed to stimulate circulation and provide energy, and the *pegaga* leaves are widely used as a supposed aphrodisiac and for a variety of ailments including asthma.

This bomoh claimed that a combination of the turmeric and ginger roots with sweet flag and *daun balik angin* is particularly useful in "strengthening the bones of the body" and making the body "regain the proper flow of oxygen." In addition to his own herbal mixtures he also prescribes *majun* and *jamun* to restore appetite and generally to "strengthen the body!" Both *majun* and *jamun* are commonly used vegetal mixtures said to be good for a variety of ailments and are sold as aphrodisiacs by a number of itinerant folk medicine peddlers. *Majun* has been known to contain Indian hemp, datura, and poppy seeds, but different recipes are in use and it is not certain that the *majun* used by this bomoh contains these ingredients. LaBarre (1975) reports the use of *majun* in India, where it is known by the same name and is supposedly "made of cannabis with sugar and spices, sometimes with added datura and opium" (p. 28).

Experiments made with two samples of the concoctions of unknown ingredients used by two of the five bomohs studied in 1978–1979 and extracts from the *buah mengkudu* were carried out on mice at the School of Pharmaceutical Sciences, Universiti

Sains Malaysia, Penang. Both the fruit and the leaves of the *mengkudu*, a common shrub in Malaysia, have been used extensively in traditional medicinal treatment for such ailments as headache, cholera, diarrhea, and various fevers. It was found that extracts from the pulp of the *buah mengkudu* (*morinda citrifolia*), when given to mice undergoing withdrawal, cause suppression of precipitated withdrawal jumping in mice, and have spasmogenic action on the smooth muscles of the guinea pig ileum (Prabhakaran 1979).

One of the bomoh samples suppressed precipitated withdrawal jumping in mice, but the sample from the second bomoh did not. Both samples had a general depressant action on mice and both caused hypothermia in mice. Although the second bomoh sample seemed to have no narcotic antagonistic property, both samples had marked analgesic effect, decreased locomotor activity, decreased exploratory behavior, and reduced spontaneous motor activity. Further studies are warranted on these and the other concoctions used by the drug bomohs, but there is little evidence that recent studies have been conducted (see for examples Arokiasamy and Taricone 1992, Lee 1985). It may be assumed, however, that the one bomoh sample and extracts from the *buah mengkudu* probably do suppress withdrawal symptoms in addicts (as well as in addicted mice) and depress their general activity (Prabhakaran 1979). It is also likely that a number of the mixtures used by other bomohs, but not tested, would produce equally effective results on close examination.

A Follow-Up Study of Addicts Treated by Malay Bomoh Healers

Because of the interest in traditional medicine, the growing problem of drug addiction in Malaysia, and the pressing need to treat and rehabilitate those dependent on drugs, a follow-up evaluation study of bomoh treatment was conducted in 1978–1979 by the author and Abdul Rashid bin Abdul Razak under the auspices of the National Drug Dependence Research Centre with the encouragement of the Malaysian Cabinet Committee on Drug Dependence (Heggenhougen 1984, 1985, Heggenhougen and Navaratnam 1979a,b). According to the literature review for this book it appears that this 1978–1979 study remains the only one to have studied this treatment alternative modality in Malaysia in some detail.

Personal, tape-recorded interviews were held with ten bomohs in the Malaysian states of Perlis, Kedah, Penang, Perak, and Selangor (Kuala Lumpur) who were actively treating heroin addicts. Some of these bomohs also saw patients for other complaints but their main healing preoccupation was as drug bomohs. Lists of names and addresses of a total of 406 addict patients treated by five of these bomohs were obtained from them in confidence. The bomohs claimed that these were the total number of patients treated by them for whom they had names and addresses. It is probable that others were treated but that their names and addresses had not been recorded. (The bomohs had started keeping records of the names and addresses of their patients several years before we had ever approached them concerning our study.) Based on intensive and repeated interviews with the bomohs one can be fairly certain that the other patients not recorded were relatively few in number and usually constituted the earliest heroin addicts treated. We were also convinced that the bomohs did not purposely withhold the names of those patients they felt were most likely to return to drug use after their treatment.

In the main part of the study an attempt was made to contact the 406 patients who had been treated by five of these healers. Intensive personal baseline and follow-up reports and urine samples were obtained for 102 of these patients; baseline but no follow-up progress interviews were held with another eight patients. Less substantial information was obtained on 122 additional patients from interviews held with their relatives, as it was impossible to contact the patients themselves. No follow-up information was available for the remaining 174 patients due to incomplete or false addresses and residence in states not visited.

The evaluation of this particular treatment modality includes a description of the treatment methods used by bomohs (Heggenhougen and Navaratnam 1979a,b), discussion of the unique methodological research problems involved, description of the patient population, rates of abstinence and other results of pharmacological tests on treatment "teas," and a discussion of the role of these healers in treating Malaysian addicts in the future. The intention was to present an overview of traditional methods of drug addiction treatment and to provide an insight into the treatment of heroin addicts in Malaysia.

The study of drug addiction is a particularly sensitive area of research both in national and in individual terms. Every effort was made to provide confidentiality to those studied and to be sensitive to national concerns and to national efforts to eliminate drug addiction and to rehabilitate those addicted. The study itself came about because of a general interest in any treatment and rehabilitation methods, no matter how unique, that might prove to be helpful to addicts, and as a result of earlier research on traditional Malaysian folk medicine carried out in association with the Malaysian Institute for Medical Research. In the course of this previous research it became known that a number of bomohs were treating addicts, and the issue of traditional treatment of addicts was a central concern of the newly formed Association of Traditional Malay Medicine. The names and locations of these folk healers were obtained from this association, and a few others became known through occasional articles about them in the local press and through conversations with bomohs and with addicts and former addicts with whom we had contact.

The bomohs' cooperation was secured, in part, through the help of the newly elected president of the Association of Traditional Malay Medicine (Heggenhougen 1979), but as the treatment methods were not officially recognized there was some hesitancy on the part of the bomohs to provide full information about the ingredients of their prescriptions. There was also some concern that their medicine, in which they showed confidence, would be appropriated and used by others, without giving them due credit.

To evaluate the effectiveness of bomoh treatment of addicts an attempt was made to contact and conduct personal interviews with each of the 406 patients. These interviews were designed to determine the progress of the patients subsequent to treatment and to establish rates of abstinence and recidivism for patients of the different bomohs. The World Health Organization (WHO)-developed baseline and progress forms were used in these interviews along with our own questionnaire for bomoh patients. Baseline interviews were held with 110 respondents of whom 102 were also interviewed using the follow-up progress forms. Urine samples were taken from all those interviewed to corroborate the responses. Most of the urine samples were analyzed by the School of Pharmaceutical Sciences at the Universiti Sains Malaysia and the rest by the Division of Biochemistry of the Institute for Medical Research, Kuala Lumpur. The WHO interview forms were coded and tabulated at the Universiti Sains Malaysia computer center.

Brief interviews about the whereabouts of former patients were held with relatives of those patients who were not at home or who had moved from the addresses provided by the bomohs. Information obtained from relatives was recorded on a one-page form. Initially, letters were mailed to the potential respondents requesting an interview appointment, but we eventually stopped doing this as we found such letters to be relatively ineffective, and we suspected that some former patients would be unavailable if they knew someone was coming to interview them. Once contacted, however, all but six former patients agreed to be interviewed and, contrary to what might have been expected, most spoke freely and at length about their current situation and past experiences.

A few parents showed reluctance in having their sons speak with the interviewer as they did not want them to be reminded of their period of drug taking, believing that this would make the respondents wish to return to drug use. When contacted, each potential respondent was requested to cooperate with the interviewer but was also told that there was no obligation for him (only one respondent is female) to do so and he was assured that there would be no negative consequences should he wish not to cooperate or to answer only some of the questions asked. Patients were also assured confidentiality and special code identification numbers were used on the interview forms rather than names.

Repeated attempts were made to obtain interviews with former patients. As the population was highly mobile, many patients could not be located at the addresses given. Attempts were also made to locate those who had moved. This search for former patients was time-consuming and required persistence.

As discussions of heroin addiction are extremely sensitive, the issue of confidentiality was emphasized. When it was impossible to locate the patients or their relatives, we inquired of their neighbors, but we did not mention drugs. The Malay interviewer/co-investigator engaged people in general conversation, which within Malay culture is a matter of polite form, before asking specific questions. Respondents, especially villagers, were found to be open about information when speaking to a fellow Malay. The former patient's previous drug addiction was often brought up by the relatives and neighbors themselves when discussing the former patient; otherwise, the subject of addiction was not raised by the interviewer. The preliminary "small talk" is time-consuming, but if a more direct approach is taken, interviewees might take offense and withhold information or refuse to cooperate.

All interviews with former patients and with relatives were carried out during the first half of 1979 by Abdul Rashid bin Abdul Razak in Malay (as most of the patients using this treatment method are Muslim Malay males under 30 years of age) and occasionally in English. The quality of a study is related to the quality of the research instruments used, and when an in-depth, detailed interview technique is used, the researcher/interviewer himself is such an "instrument." The character of the interviewer and the manner in which he introduces himself and relates to the interviewee are particularly important with as sensitive a subject as drug addiction. The interviewer, who represented the backbone of this study, is particularly qualified in a number of ways:

1. He is a Muslim, as are most of the patients we tried to contact, and thus he shares the cultural background of these patients.
2. He has lived for extensive periods in both village and inner-city urban settings. He is familiar with the drug scene (through friends and relatives and through having lived near "copping areas"), although he himself has never been involved in drug taking. The rural/urban combination is important in that this is often the experience of the addicts themselves. There is often a conflict between rural and urban values, between traditional and more cosmopolitan ways of behavior. The interviewer bridges these worlds.

3. The interviewer is a former customs officer who has worked on the Malaysian/Thai border and has himself apprehended drug smugglers.
4. Previous to his involvement in this project he worked for more than two years as a research assistant with the Malaysian Institute for Medical Research on projects concerning rural health and traditional medicine. He is thus familiar with the practices of folk healers and has had extensive training and experience in interviewing bomohs and their patients.
5. He is not a university graduate and does not intimidate the addicts with a sense of superiority or distance; however, his ability to empathize with those he interviews, making them feel at ease, is combined with a sense of authority and assurance.

Many of the former addicts interviewed had used a number of different resources in their attempts to overcome their addiction. This presented a methodological problem. The patient of a particular bomoh might be free from drugs at follow-up, but the credit could not be given to the bomoh's treatment if the patient had subsequently returned to drugs and then attended another treatment program. In such instances we recorded that this bomoh's patient returned to drug taking and noted the elapsed period of time. It is somewhat difficult to detect this multiple treatment utilization from the WHO forms, but the responses to our additional questionnaire record the different treatments. Notes were taken of additional open-ended discussions with the respondents during which a number of issues were raised. We decided to attribute credit for drug-free patients to the most recent treatment, even though it might well be that the combination of treatments, rather than the most recent treatment alone, was responsible for abstinence.

This was a limited, retrospective study, but we feel that valuable information is provided in an area of addiction treatment about which little is known. Although we cannot speak in definitive or comparative terms, the results show that this treatment method has validity. Future comprehensive and more detailed studies, for which our study serves as a useful beginning, would be fruitful. The treatment methodology we attempted to evaluate is highly unique. The bomohs operate on an individual basis and most treat only a few addicts at a time. Thus, to interview more than just a few patients, we obtained a list of all the former addict patients for whom the five bomohs had names and addresses. Some of these former addict patients had been treated more than a year ago, whereas others had been seen more recently; the average time since treatment of all those interviewed was a little over 12 months.

There may have been a possible effect of the interviews themselves. As mentioned, a number of parents did not want their children to be interviewed because they felt this would recall the days of drug taking that they wanted their children to forget. This attitude should not be treated lightly. We must also keep in mind that a substantial number of former patients are younger than 21 and live at home, and the majority of all patients had used heroin before the age of 20.

Elsewhere it has been discussed that one of the potential factors influencing former addicts to return to drugs is a sudden association or reminder of past drug-taking activity (Lex and Meyer 1977, Winkler 1974a,b). We point this out to warn of the hazards of this type of research and to emphasize the necessity for tactfulness and caution on the part of the interviewer. The research presents a dilemma: on the one hand, we would like to obtain sufficient data on enough former patients to make the study worthwhile and of use in guiding future treatment/ rehabilitation programs so as to benefit other addicts or potential addicts; on the other hand, we need to consider the sensitivity of the research and to guard against any negative effect of the process of the research itself.

As verified by urine sample analysis, half of the patients interviewed were abstinent at the time of the interview—an average of twelve months after treatment. We therefore cannot assume that bomoh treatment results in an abstinence rate as high as 50 percent a year after treatment, however, since the rate for those not interviewed might be lower. If we make the worst-case assumption that all those not interviewed had returned to drug use, the abstinence rate of patients treated by these five bomohs would then be 13 percent. Thus, we can assume an abstinence rate of 13 to 50 percent. However, the worst-case average abstinence rate for patients of two of the bomohs is approximately 30 percent a year after treatment, because for these two bomohs the abstinence rate of the patients we did interview was better than 65 percent (Heggenhougen and Navaratnam 1979b)—certainly better than abstinence rates achieved by orthodox programs.

The following six tables summarize the results for the 102 patients of all bomohs (Table 2–1) and for the patients of each of the five bomohs (Tables 2–2 through 2–6).

TABLE 2–1. Drug-taking status of 102 of the 406 patients of the five bomohs interviewed

	Bomoh treatment only	Bomoh as last treatment	Bomoh neither last nor first	Bomoh first of several	Other	Total
Non-drug free after bomoh treatment	6	10	26	7	4	53 (52%)
Non-drug free now	6	10	12	1	3	32
Drug free after bomoh treatment	18	27	1	–	3	49 (48%)
Drug free now	18	27	15	6	4	70
Total	24	37	27	7	7	102

TABLE 2–2. Drug-taking status of 23 of the 46 patients of Bomoh A interviewed

	A's treatment only	A as last treatment	A neither last nor first	A first of several	Other	Total
Non-drug free after A treatment	1	1	3[1]	3	2	10
Non-drug free now	1	1	1[1]	–	1	4
Drug free after A treatment	7	6	–	–	–	13 (56.5%)
Drug free now	7	6	2[1]	3	1	19 (82.6%)
Total	8 (14.7 mo.)	7 (13.5 mo.)	3[1] (15.6 mo.)	3 (22.6 mo.)	2 (14.5 mo.)	23 (15.5 mo.)

[1]Urine tests were negative for all three patients but interviewer suspects at least one of these to be back on drugs. One claimed he did not return to drug use but wanted other treatment "to be sure," another said he became addicted to the bomoh's "tea." All three are here recorded as having returned to drug use after Bomoh A's treatment.

TABLE 2–3. Drug-taking status of 27 of the 67 patients of Bomoh B interviewed

	B's treatment only	B as last treatment	B neither last nor first	B first of several	Other	Total
Non-drug free after B treatment	–	1	3	4	–	8
Non-drug free now	–	1	2	1	–	4
Drug free after B treatment	8[1]	10[2]	–	–	1	19 (67%)
Drug free now	8[1]	10	1	3	1	23
Total	8[1] (8.3 mo.)	11 (11.1 mo.)	3 (18 mo.)	4 (18.8 mo.)	1 (17 mo.)	27 (12.6 mo.)

[1]One of these still takes the bomoh's "tea" (five months after treatment), and the wife of another claims he is taking opium chips (but urine tests were negative for all eight).
[2]One still takes the bomoh's "tea" (three months after treatment); one tried the bomoh's treatment three different times (and relapsed), but he has now finally managed to be off drugs for the past 19 months "as a result of" the bomoh's treatment.

TABLE 2–4. Drug-taking status of 3 of the 66 patients of Bomoh C interviewed

	C's treatment only	C as last treatment	C neither last nor first	C first of several	Other	Total
Non-drug free after C treatment	–	–	1	–	–	1 (33.3%)
Non-drug free now	–	–	1	–	–	1
Drug free after C treatment	1	1	–	–	–	2 (66.7%)
Drug free now	1	1	–	–	–	2
Total	1	1	1	–	–	3

TABLE 2–5. Drug-taking status of 40 of the 183 patients of Bomoh D interviewed

	D's treatment only	D as last treatment	D neither last nor first	D first of several	Other	Total
Non-drug free after D treatment	3^1	$6^{1,2}$	17^7	–	2^8	28 (70%)
Non-drug free now	3	6	8^6	–	2	19 (47.5%)
Drug free after D treatment	2	$8^{3,4,5}$	–	–	2	12 (30%)
Drug free now	2	8	9	–	2^9	21 (52.5%)
Total	5 (13.8 mo.)	14 (12.4 mo.)	17 (12.8 mo.)	–	4 (10.5 mo.)	40 (12.6 mo.)

[1] One did not give urine sample but was judged relapsed by interviewer.
[2] The interviewer had not suspected that two of these were relapsed but urine test was positive.
[0] Three of these claimed the bomoh's treatment was ineffective even though they have not relapsed. They gave credit to their own rather than to the bomoh's efforts.
[4] One had just been detoxified at a rehabilitation center but went to the bomoh to get a "hatred charm."
[5] One of these might be beginning to relapse as he has taken drugs a few times since treatment.
[6] One had tried as many as ten different treatments; another had tried eight.
[7] Three had later been treated successfully by another bomon, three by a rehabilitation center, two by a hospital, and one attributed current abstinence to his own self-treatment.
[8] There was no urine sample for one of these, but he was judged relapsed by the interviewer.
[9] The interviewer had judged these two as relapsed but urine tests were negative. It is not known if these sought other treatment after bomoh treatment; thus it is not absolutely certain these abstained because of bomoh D's treatment.

TABLE 2–6. Drug-taking status of 9 of the 44 patients of Bomoh E interviewed

	E's treatment only	E as last treatment	E neither last nor first	E first of several	Other	Total
Non-drug free after E treatment	2^1	2^2	2	–	–	6 (66 2/3%)
Non-drug free now	2	2	–	–	–	4
Drug free after E treatment	–	2	1^3	–	–	3 (33 1/3%)
Drug free now	–	2	3	–	–	5
Total	2 (5.5 mo.)	4 (9.3 mo.)	3 (10 mo.)	–	–	9 (8.7 mo.)

[1] The interviewer had not expected that one of these was back on drugs but urine was positive.
[2] There was no urine sample for one of these but patient told interviewer he was taking drugs.
[3] The patient did not relapse after E's treatment but spent one month as an inpatient in a hospital psychiatric ward immediately after the bomoh's treatment.

3

Buddhist and Traditional Medical Therapies of Addicts in Thailand

> It has been a natural evolution for the Buddhist temple to assume the role of treatment centre in response to the growth of drug dependence.... The temple can be regarded as providing the genuine indigenous treatment of drug dependence in Thailand.
>
> Poshyachinda 1980

> Most men enter priesthood for a period before marriage.... This tradition was extended to the ordination of delinquent offsprings with the belief that the life and teaching of the temple will reform their conduct.
>
> Poshyachinda 1993

Opium and heroin addicts have been treated in a number of Buddhist temples in Thailand for decades (Heggenhougen 1984, 1985, Jilek-Aall and Jilek 1985, Poshyachinda 1980, 1982, 1984, 1993, Suwanwela and Poshyachinda 1983, 1986). Some of the monks involved in these temple therapies have been trained at the Centre for Traditional Thai Buddhist Medicine at Wat Pho (Pho Temple) in Bangkok, where people can come for treatment of a range of ailments or for a genuine massage. Traditional healers have had an association with the Buddhist temples throughout Thailand, especially as healing is seen to be an integrated process involving spiritual as well as physical and psychosocial interventions. Many of the country's healers practice and see their patients within a temple setting and have done so for centuries, treating patients for the full range of ailments with which they are afflicted. The setting of the temple and the spiritual component of treatment tend to add to the confidence patients have in these healers even though outsiders can sometimes be skeptical about the healers' therapeutic claims.

It would be interesting to do a follow-up study on the patients of Phra (Rev.) Preeja Ativatano of the Institute of Resurrection, Wat Paapoen, Chiang Mai Province, who in 1978 appeared overly optimistic when claiming to be able to treat "cancer, hemorrhoids, adenoids, asthma, gastritis, neurasthenia, high and low blood pressure, heart disease, tuberculosis, gall-stones, provide psychotherapy, epilepsy, diabetes and all kinds of narcotic addiction" (Preeja 1978). But despite one's initial impulse to characterize such encompassing claims as nonsense, some of the interventions used may be effective. Like many of his colleagues elsewhere, Phra Preeja began to treat opium and heroin addicts at the end of the 1960s; some traditional Thai healers had treated opium addicts long before that. Phra Preeja gave his addict patient an herbal concoction that causes vomiting and convulsions to the extent that the patient needed to be tied down during the first day of treatment. The patient stayed at the temple for only a few days and was given a different herbal mixture to take at home whenever he felt a craving for drugs. The ingredients of these concoctions were kept secret.

Wat Soda, another Chiang Mai temple visited in 1978, is within the "Golden Triangle" and served as a rehabilitation center not because addicts were given special treatment there but because many addicts who had been detoxified by government programs joined the priesthood and became monks there for various periods of time—some for several years—to strengthen their resolve to stay away from drugs, to develop a positive identity, and to gain coping skills when reentering the world outside the temple compound. North of Chiang Mai, in Fang near the Burmese border, Phra Mahawan Sira Wongse treated addicts at an abandoned temple where he kept them for five days of detoxification with herbal tablets. Other such temples included Wat Pay Pang in Chiang Mai, Tam Talu Centre in Ratchaburi, and Wat Tha Shee Srisumungklaran in Roi-et provinces. Each temple treated addicts in a slightly different way but usually involved a combination of an herbal detoxification mixture with spiritual lessons, general counseling, and skills training. By the 1980s, however, it was primarily only Wat Soda and Wat Tam Kramborg that continued such addiction therapies.

The most well known of the temples where addicts have been treated and rehabilitated is the Wat Tam Kraborg, 130 kilometers northeast of Bangkok, which started addiction therapy in 1963. All patients had to volunteer for treatment and were treated only once. No one was given a second chance. Upon entrance into the program all addicts made a vow to the Buddha concerning their sincerity and determination to be cured and to stay away from drugs following treatment. An herbal medicine, which produced vomiting and sweating, was given for five days during the withdrawal/detoxification period—the purging period—followed by five days of rest and recuperation—the strengthening period. The addicts were treated together in large groups by the charismatic Abbot Phra Chamroon Pauchand and in addition to the medicine received formal counseling and Buddhist religious lessons. The temple had four rules:

- complete abstinence from drugs causing dependence
- obedience to the priest
- no disruptive behavior
- remain within the temple compound throughout the treatment period without any excuses.

> [The treatment proper constituted various] combination[s] of religious rite, herbal medicine, moral counselling, religious teaching and vocational training. The Wat Soda used [a] funeral ceremony to initiate the treatment process. The clients carried out a mock funeral cremating their own evil self that depended on drugs. The ceremony implied the rebirth of a new clean life.... The Wat Tam Kramborg had herbal steam bath supplement to the herbal medicine and a range of optional vocational training in agricultural work, garment manufacturing and car repair. [Poshyachinda 1993, p. 3]

Again at the completion of the ten days of treatment each patient had to swear to the Buddha in front of the abbot not to return to drug use. Many of the treated patients became apprenticed monks for a certain time and others were ordained as priests, thus serving in the temple for a considerable period.

The herbal therapy used in detoxification was first developed by a Buddhist nun, an herbalist, from Saraburi Province, whose compassion and desire to help opium addicts led her to experiment with various herbal mixtures. The result was the special herbal therapy used at Wat Tam Kramborg. She instructed her nephew, the present abbot Phra Chamroon Paruchan, about the mixture and he refined the therapy further and developed the systematic therapeutic approach that was used in the treatment of more than 50,000 addicts until the government, for unknown reasons, prohibited the temple from continuing such addiction therapy in the early 1990s. By 1975, however, when the temple had used its particular approach to treat many thousands of addicts for twelve years, the abbot was awarded the International Mag Sai Award for public service (Poshyachinda 1993).

A preliminary follow-up evaluation of 1,054 patients treated at Wat Tam Kraborg from October 1976 through February 1977 showed that from 70 to 80 percent of the heroin addicts returned

Buddhist and Traditional Therapies in Thailand 39

to drug use after six months and close to 90 percent were recidivists one year after treatment. However, only slightly more than 40 percent of the opium addicts treated had returned to drug use six months after treatment. The results are based on a mail survey of patients at three, six, and twelve months following treatment, with a total of 43 percent responding at least once. Although the validity of the mail response was checked by a random intensive follow-up sampling, including urine testing of 4 percent of the total, this, as stated by the authors, "does not pretend to be a scientific report on an evaluation research" (Poshyachinda et al. 1978, p. 3). But this study and Westermeyer's studies are a beginning, and they throw some light on this type of treatment modality. Another study showed "the abstinence rate six months after discharge for the heroin users from Bangkok was about 20% and for those from the provincial cities about 30%" (Poshyachinda 1980, p. 124).

The recidivism rates for patients of government and private clinics were 55 to 70 percent for opium addicts and 95 to 100 percent for heroin users. Thus, government heroin treatment simply meant addicts could lower their heroin requirements, and thus their expenses, for a few months subsequent to treatment.

> The extensive service provided over many years by the Wat Tam Kraborg gradually changed the temple into a new kind of therapeutic religious institution that no longer carried the image and religious atmosphere of a Buddhist temple.
> ... The most apparent changes over these long years was the gradual disappearance of the valuable therapeutic environment of peace and the non-verbal expression of care between all parties concerned. These changes were perhaps partly responsible for the downward drift of the statistical decline in abstinence efficacy. [Poshyachinda 1993, p. 11]

4
Other Traditional and Herbal Therapies

> [The] application of the herbal [made from the seeds of the "haba de San Ignacio" (*Hura polyandra L.*)] and a similar application of a few other remedios, are in common use as one form of indigenous alcohol therapy on the Eastern portion of the United States–Mexico border.
>
> Trotter 1979

As discussed in the previous chapters, herbs, either singly or in combination, are often central to alternative addiction therapies. Herbs are not usually relied on alone; they are used primarily during the withdrawal and detoxification stage of therapy. At times herbal mixtures are also used to create an aversion to alcohol and addictive drugs. Unlike methadone, however, the great majority of the herbal mixtures used to treat addicts are taken for a limited period and do not themselves lead to addiction. "Next to opium, valerian root, the major ingredients in 'relaxo brew' is nature's best sedative, and it is nonaddicting" (Nebelkopf 1987, p. 704).

Nebelkopf (1987, 1988) reports the use of herbs in different parts of the world, such as in the detoxification of addicted Lao hill tribe refugees in Thailand; in the Nuevo Amanecer program in Colombia, a residential therapeutic community for adolescent drug abusers that uses herbs in a natural approach to drug rehabilitation; and in addiction therapies in North America. "The first publication concerning herbal treatment in the context of a free clinic was *Healing Yourself*, a self-help manual published by the Country Doctor Free Clinic in Seattle" (Nebelkopf 1988, p. 350).

> White Bird Sociomedical Aid Station, a free clinic in Eugene, Oregon, developed a comprehensive alternative health care system, integrating traditional medical care with innovative approaches, such as herbs and acupuncture, in a pioneering attempt to deal with the whole person in the context of a self-help approach. [Nebelkopf 1988, p. 351]

> The Lincoln Detoxification Program at Lincoln Hospital in New York City pioneered the utilization of herbal therapy in conjunction with acupuncture in a natural healing approach to drug detoxification. In this program, skullcap, hops and valerian were used as nervines, golden seal and dandelion were used to improve liver function, and alfalfa provided a wide variety of vitamins, minerals and digestive enzymes. . . . [In] the 3HO Program in Tucson, Arizona . . . clients receive massages and hot baths to promote relaxation, eat a well-balanced vegetarian diet and participate in a daily schedule of yoga. . . . [The program] utilizes a wide variety of herbs, including cayenne and golden seal, beet juice (an excellent blood purifier) and Yogi Tea, which consists of ginger, cinnamon, cloves, cardamom and peppercorns. [p. 352]

> By choosing such healing plants as comfrey, golden seal, mullein, ginseng, and valerian root, the substance abuser can begin to explore a healthier and more natural life-style. . . . On the other hand, there are herbal stimulants which do not contain caffeine (ginseng, gotu kola, sassafras, sarsaparilla) but which do have stimulant effects on the ner-

vous and circulatory systems without the negative effects of caffeine. [Nebelkopf 1987, pp. 699, 702]

Ayurvedic herbal mixtures have been used for a considerable time against addiction in a number of settings in India and elsewhere in Asia and a recent study by Shanmugasundaram and Shanmugasundaram (1986) tested one such mixture and concluded that "it appears to be a promising way to combat alcoholism" (p. 171).

As has been mentioned earlier (see Chapter 2), Chinese herbal medicines have also been used for a considerable time to treat opium addicts. Yang and colleagues (1985) studied the use of such herbs by 300 addict patients in Hong Kong.

> Chinese herbs were used in the treatment of opium and heroin addicts in Hong Kong. The results of three hundred cases were analyzed and evaluated. . . . The herbs *Qiang Huo, Gou Teng, Chuan Ziong, Fu Zi* and *Yan Hu Suo* were found to reduce the three main withdrawal scores significantly. . . .
>
> After 2 years' follow-up observation, it was found that the successful rate was 48%. . . . Some of the patients reported that during the treatment they refused to take opium or heroin again because they suffered nausea and even vomiting upon smelling such drugs. . . . Chinese herbal medicine was helpful in overcoming their craving for drugs. . . . Sometimes, acupuncture treatment was supplemented and the combination treatment was considered better than the single one. [Yang et al. 1985, pp. 147–148]

Traditional healers (*curanderos*) in Latin America and in the southern United States are also called upon to treat alcoholics and many use special herbs in so doing. Concerning the use of such treatment for alcoholics along the United States/

Mexican border Trotter (1979) reported on the use of a specific seed called,

> "Haba de San Ignacio" (*Hura plyandra L.* and *Hura crepitans L.*) to promote an aversion to the consumption of alcohol by problem drinkers in Mexican American and Mexican national populations on the United States–Mexico border....
>
> Individuals are instructed to prepare the seed by roasting it well on a comal or griddle until it is thoroughly cooked. The covering is peeled from the cooled seed and the meat of the seed is placed in a mocajete (mortar and pestle), then ground into a fine powder. This powder is placed in food or drink that will be consumed by the person with the alcohol problem.... The problem drinker is normally given the remedy without his or her knowledge; however, on at least two occasions curanderos stated they had used the herbal with the patient's knowledge, when the drinker, rather than a relative, had asked for help in eliminating a drinking problem....
>
> When the individual... consumes alcohol later in the day or the evening, he becomes nauseated, vomits, and may have some diarrhea.... Often the therapy works as intended, to form an aversion to alcohol.... Sometimes this remedio works, and the man stops drinking; but other times he just stops coming home for dinner. [pp. 279, 281]

Ibogaine

Recently, a great deal of attention in Europe and in the United States has been given to the use and study of the herb ibogaine (*Tabernathe iboga*), a flowering shrub native to West Africa, originally used in healing and revitalization ceremonies by the Bwiti Cult in Gabon (Fernandez 1972). Ibogaine apparently interacts with dopamine, a neurotransmitter that plays a key role in addiction. The use of this herb has been discussed both in the popular press, such as *Newsweek* and the *New York Times Magazine*, as well as in the scientific literature. According to the *New York Times* article,

> It halts drug cravings for months and sometimes years without inducing withdrawal. It unleashes a 36-hour slide show of buried memories that jars addicts into reassessing their drug-ravaged lives. Finally, unlike methadone and other narcotic substitutes, it suppresses the desire for hard drugs without creating another dependency. . . . Researchers believe ibogaine interacts with dopamine, the neurotransmitter that plays a key role in addiction. [Jester 1994, pp. 50, 52]

The *Newsweek* article (Cowley et al. 1993) discussed its use for a number of years by Howard Lotsof in his addiction treatment program in the Netherlands; he has now submitted a patent application in the United States for its use under the brand name of Endabuse. A large trial to test ibogaine in 300 volunteers addicted to heroin and cocaine is presently being conducted in the Netherlands.

Articles in the scientific journals also report on ibogaine's reputed efficacy, for example in the *Journal of NIH Research*:

> After a three-day trip, they apparently found that ibogaine ended their craving for heroin, cocaine, and other illicit drugs for several months to years. . . . The drug . . . may be an effective treatment for addiction to cocaine, heroin, amphetamines, and perhaps to alcohol and nicotine. . . . Lotsof has been administering ibogaine to volunteer addicts in The Netherlands over the past five years. Sisko says that with the exception of one woman who died of a heroin overdose while taking ibogaine, all have kicked their drug

habit for between three months to several years. [Touchette 1993, pp. 50, 51]

Because of the mounting anecdotal evidence on the power of ibogaine a number of scientific studies are now being undertaken, and preliminary results have been promising (Cappendijk and Dzoljic 1993, Deecher et al. 1992, Glick et al. 1991, Maisonneuve and Glick 1992). Again, from the *Journal of NIH Research*:

> [Glick] reported in 1991 that, on average, a single injection of ibogaine, administered before or after morphine, decreased morphine intake by nearly 50% a day after administration and by 30 to 40% for up to a week after administration. . . . A single ibogaine injection decreased cocaine intake by 40 to 60% for several days, and . . . repeated ibogaine administration at one-week intervals produced 60 to 80% decreases in cocaine intake that lasted for several weeks. . . .
>
> One of the most intriguing aspects of ibogaine is its apparent ability . . . to end addiction and drug craving in humans without inducing withdrawal symptoms. . . . Another unanswered question is whether ibogaine has different effects in males and females. Lotsof says that in his experiences, ibogaine seems more effective in females. . . . "People are going overseas to get this treatment" says Curtis Wright of FDA. "If this is an efficacious treatment for drug addiction, we need to know this soon. If it's harmful, we need to know that sooner." [Touchette 1993, pp. 52, 55]

5

Native American Therapies in the United States

> Revived traditional Amerindian ceremonials, redefined and adjusted to the therapeutic needs of the younger generation, are successful in combating alcoholism among certain aboriginal peoples of North America.
>
> Jilek 1993a

A range of traditional Native American healing, revitalization, and *rite de pasage* (death and rebirth rite of passage) rituals have been adapted by Native American people for the purpose of treating the disproportionately high number of Native American alcoholics and other drug addicts in North America. There is growing evidence of their effectiveness (Howard 1976, Jilek 1978, 1989, 1993a,b). Even when the primary declared purpose is not to treat addicts but rather to confirm a positive identity, support a vision quest, and strengthen, develop, and mature the participants, the revival of dance and revitalization rituals has had an ancillary preventive impact as well as a positive effect on those already addicted and has inhibited, and often completely eliminated, addictive behavior. The therapeutic practices based on traditional healing ceremonies are increasingly used to treat Native American alcoholics and are being shown to be more effective than standard rehabilitation programs.

The cross-cultural psychiatrist Jilek (1978, 1989, 1993a,b) has written extensively on the resurgence and the efficacy of Native American therapeutic ceremonials. Others have also produced significant evidence that these ceremonies have both prophylactic as well as therapeutic efficacy. The rituals can be considered rites of passage from a less to a more preferred state and often involves "transformation and retransformation; fragmentation and reassemblage; infection (or intrusion) and catharsis; separation and reunification" (Jilek 1978, p. 119).

> These [North American] indigenous group therapeutic endeavors use altered states of consciousness and are especially geared to the effective treatment and prevention of alcohol and drug dependence, cultural change-related dysthymic conditions (anomic depression) and psychosomatic disorders. Examples are the Sun Dance ceremonial of Amerindian tribes in Wyoming, Idaho, Utah, Colorado, North and South Dakota; the Winter Spirit Dance of the Salish Indians in British Columbia and Washington State, and the medicine societies of the Iroquois Indians in Canada and New York State.... The general conclusion to be drawn from these reports is that the above cited traditional group therapies involving altered states of consciousness are subjectively and objectively effective methods of symptom removal, restoration of functioning and social rehabilitation, in the following conditions: 1) neurotic-reactive syndromes such as anxiety states, dysthymia, "hysterical" somatiform and "functional" psychophysiologic disorders; 2) reactive and anomic depression; and 3) alcohol and drug dependence. [Jilek 1993a, p. 354]

The *Gourd Dance* of the Plains Indians is one of these ceremonies that now involves a number of groups such as the Navajo,

Cree, Blackfoot, and Ojibwa, and is credited with rehabilitating many of the participants who were alcoholics (Jilek 1989).

> Besides the aspects of ego strengthening, group support, and meaningful collective activity, gourd dance societies afford their members opportunities for socially sanctioned and approved abreactions. As a gourd dance session progresses, excitement builds during special "fast songs" played toward the end of the ceremony when drumming and rattling tempo increase to culminate in psychodramatic discharges of aggressive feelings. [Jilek 1978, p. 132]

The *Sun Dance* originated with the Plains Algonquians 300 years ago and shifted from being related to hunting to being used in treating illness. The participants dance for three to four days and nights, during which time they are deprived of food and drink and they sustain various degrees of mutilation ("tearing the flesh"). The Sun Dance was revitalized in the 1950s and by the 1960s had more followers than the Native American Church (NAC). The experiences of altered states of consciousness (ASC), similar to those occurring in shamanic initiation ceremonies and during the personal vision quests that were part of a traditional past, were induced by the dance, and are central mechanisms of therapeutic efficacy. The preparation for and participation in the Sun Dance constitute a profound teaching experience for most of the participants.

> There is identity and ego-strengthening significance in such teaching for many a culturally drifting young Amerindian person whose self-esteem has been undermined by experiences in the majority society. . . . In entering an altered state of consciousness . . . [the participant] is helped by intensive rhythmic drumming. . . . Specific shamanizing

curing rites [are also incorporated and adds to the] psychosociotherapeutic function of the Sun Dance. [Jilek 1989, pp. 174–175]

The *Winter Spirit Dance* of the Native Americans along the Pacific Coast involves spirit singing and dancing.

The major purpose of continuing participation in the annual winter dances is to strengthen the self-healing power and to maintain a wholesome state of mind and body . . . [and participants now also include] young Amerindians with behavioral, alcohol, and drug problems, as candidates for spirit dance initiation. [Jilek 1989, p. 168]

During an initiation period of from four to ten days, the candidate has to endure psychological stress, seclusion, and restricted mobility in a dark smokehouse cubicle; this alternates with periods of forced hypermobility, visual-sensory and sleep deprivation, and kinetic, tactile, pain, and temperature stimulation.

The treatment aims at the depatterning of the faulty old personality under the combined effect of psychophysiological measures and collective and individual suggestions. Such depatterning paves the way for reorientation toward the ideal norms of native culture through a comprehensive program of indoctrination and group exercises. [Jilek 1978, p. 138]

The personality depatterning is facilitated by the participant entering into trance states or altered states of consciousness produced and enhanced by drumming and dancing. The process ends with the participants' disrobing, which symbolizes discarding the previous self and the taking on of a new personality. Jilek (1989) suggests that a number of somatopsychological factors are present in all of these healing rituals that help to produce the altered states of consciousness central to the conversion of the alcoholic. These include

- rhythmic acoustic stimulation
- kinetic stimulation
- forced hypermobility
- hyperventilation
- pain stimulation
- temperature stimulation
- dehydration and hypoglycemia
- sleep deprivation
- visual-sensory deprivation
- seclusion and restricted mobility.

Jilek (1989) goes on to state that "some of the known therapeutic results observed in traditional ceremonials could be due to the antidysphoric, mood-elevating, and anxiolytic effects of endogenous opioids released in the course of these ritual procedures." However, he makes the further point that the positive change and therapeutic personality strengthening processes that occur also "result from the skillful manipulation of culturally validated symbols" (pp. 182–183).

Native American Church—Peyote Rituals

Many of the rituals involved do not include the ingestion of special foods or other substances; rather, fasting is often prescribed. However, a special form of the Native American rituals involves the ritual use of peyote. Among others, this is a special feature of the all-night religious ceremonies of the Native American Church (NAC) that have taken place for decades. The relationship between reduction of alcoholism and participation in therapeutic peyote rituals through the NAC or other ceremonies has been noted and continues to be confirmed (Roy 1973). Two decades ago Albaugh and Anderson (1974) stated, "We do not propose that either the pharmacological effects of peyote or the NAC by itself is a cure for alcoholism. . . . The NAC does, however, seem to offer some specific advantages in the treatment of the unique problems of Indian alcoholics; others have reported success in the treatment of alcoholism in Indian populations by NAC alone" (p. 1249).

Also Bergman (1971) stated,

> The NAC of North America is a religious group of Indian people of almost all tribes who believe that the hallucinogenic cactus plant peyote (*Lophophora williamsii*) is a God-given sacrament and who eat significant amounts of it during religious ceremonies. . . . The meetings are held in the home of one of the participating families . . . [and] begins at sunset and ends at sunrise. . . . After a certain point in the service, peyote is passed around the circle of worshipers and each is free to take whatever amount he wishes. . . . Much of the night is spent in the singing of religious songs. [pp. 51–52]

By 1970 the Navajo membership of the NAC numbered 40,000, 75% of whom participated in regular peyote ceremonies twice a month. The all-night ceremony is completed by a major meal in the morning during which time all participants stay together until the drug effects wear off. According to Karl Menninger (as quoted by Bergman 1971) "'Peyote is not harmful to these people; it is beneficial, comforting, inspiring, and appears to be spiritually nourishing. It is a better antidote to alcohol than anything the missionaries, the white man, and the AMA, and the public health services have come up with'" (p. 55).

Recognizing the efficacy of this ceremony the United States Public Health Service Hospital in Clinton, Oklahoma "incorporated peyote treatment into its alcoholic service program" (Blum et al. 1977, p. 460; see also Pascarosa and Futterman 1976). Blum and colleagues reported that a number of conservative non-Indian farmers (who had no "kind words for the counterculture") also participated and were helped with their alcohol problems through ritualistic/ceremonial use of peyote.

Hill (1990) notes that the use of peyote to treat alcoholism started considerably earlier than the recent rejuvenation of the Native American Church, and the other Native American revitalization ceremonies in the 1950s and 1960s. As early as 1903 the Winnebago people of Nebraska, for whom alcoholism had risen to alarming proportions at the turn of the century, used it as an antidote to alcohol. The use of peyote for other, non-alcoholic-related therapy, goes even further back in history in its use by Native American healers in their healing rituals when peyote was used ". . . to intensify the therapeutic experience and enhance the patient's insights" (Pascarosa and Futterman 1976, p. 215).

Among the Winnebago the all-night ceremonies included singing of religious songs, praying, and meditating, as well as eating peyote; the members considered themselves Christian and confessed sins openly. Confession by an alcoholic also received "social support from individuals who were closest to him socially" (Hill 1990, p. 258). By the 1930s the influence of peyotism receded and alcoholism among the Winnebago again increased. It is only with the recent rejuvenation in the use of peyote by the NAC and through other non–peyote-related ceremonies elsewhere that Native American alcoholism is again being tackled successfully.

Hill (1990) suggests that "carefully controlled studies have not demonstrated that treatment regimens for heavy drinking that use mescaline or other psychedelic drugs are any more effective than treatment approaches without them. [However,] the fire, songs, drummings, speeches, and testimonials all united with the psychoactive elements to make the experience a vivid and memorable one" (p. 259).

At least three factors are significant in the therapeutic peyote rituals: (1) the use of an official guide or "Roadman," (2) the all-night sessions that usually include singing and drumming (conducted by the "Drumman"), and (3) the use of peyote. "The Roadman defines the Indian way ('this peyote way') and 'that other way.' Guilt is mobilized as well as self-esteem strengthened [and] . . . meditative processes that lead to transpersonal consciousness are [also] encouraged" (Pascarosa and Futterman 1976, pp. 216, 218). Strict discipline is also adhered to during the all-night ceremonies.

Some have argued that the effectiveness of the peyote rituals is due to the hallucinogenic alkaloids and to the isoguinole alkaloids in the peyote, yet others have countered that it is rather the goal-directed therapeutic process that is the most decisive factor. This argument is furthered by the demonstration of the rehabilitative efficacy of the various dance ceremonials that do not require ingestion of peyote or other hallucinogenic substances. It must be noted, however, that these other ceremonies do bring about altered states of consciousness by other means and that this is central to rehabilitation.

Part of the reason for young Native Americans becoming alcoholics stems from their having entered into a limbo situation of being alienated from their own culture through so-called Westernization (not unlike the situation of young Malays in Malaysia—see Chapter 2). Without being full and equal members of the society at large, they have become strangers in their own land, which explains the effectiveness of a therapeutic process that engages the patient participant in a symbolic death and rebirth ritual that creates a new positive personality and reconfirms a solid cultural identity. This process is enhanced by the use of peyote on the one hand and by the experiences of ASC induced by the dance ceremonials on the other. They counteract isolation and alienation.

Ritualistic rites-of-passage therapeutic approaches have also taken hold among non–Native American alcoholics and drug addicts in the United States:

> We have come to the realization that for many addicts the ritual and the ceremony of "fixing" is as important as getting high. It is the Rite of Passage, the forgetting of the past, and the temporary change in one's state of mind, that is so appealing to this particular group.... The Ritual of Detoxification project was developed to provide the ritualistic heroin addict with a place and time where he can go through another [different] ceremony. [Roman 1977, p. 357]

Zinberg and colleagues (1975), in trying to understand how peyote and other hallucinogenic substances have been used for centuries without negative addictive effects by Native American groups, whereas alcohol has been misused and become addictive, explored the possibility of controlled use of potentially (but according to them not inevitably) addictive substances.

> We have established that drug subcultures can provide rituals and sanctions which limit and control use.... [A] system of social control, similar to the social control over alcohol, is a viable alternative to prohibition for minimizing drug abuse.
> The goal of these changes is not to encourage drug use. It is to remove the deviant status of controlled users so that they are susceptible to the moderating, limiting, and powerful influence of social sanctions. [Zinberg et al. 1975, pp. 180–181]

Blum and Tilton (1981) as well as McPeake and colleagues (1991), among others, suggest that achieving altered states of consciousness is a pan-human desire and that periodic experiences of ASC can be immensely beneficial. Yet, according to McPeake and colleagues (1991), "Our culture makes little provision for such experiences other than through the use of alcohol.... The need to alter one's state of consciousness emerges developmentally in children and some of their play, such as spinning to dizziness or holding their breath, is specifically designed to produce nonordinary consciousness" (p. 76). These authors argue that the failure of standard rehabilitation programs is linked to the failure, for a variety of different reasons, to address this universal human motive, whereas Native American rehabilitative therapeutic ceremonials succeed precisely because attaining ASC is incorporated into the therapeutic process.

According to Blum and Tilton (1981):

> In today's psychedelic world, loneliness and alienation are commonplace. Where love, compassion and friendship are lacking, there is always synthetic chemistry to turn you on to synthetic "high." In whatever way happiness is sought, whether through other people, drugs or sugar-coated placebos, the end result is that an individual strives in his own way to achieve happiness. [pp. 266, 269]

McPeake and colleagues (1991) describe an altered states of consciousness therapy (ASCT) program that attempts "to teach patients to consciously manipulate affect and cognition to achieve a new consciousness." They also point out that this process is basic to the approach fostered by Alcoholics Anonymous, which "clearly directs its members toward an altered state of consciousness ... a change in 'consciousness and being' called a 'spiritual awakening.' By demonstrating to patients that the same thoughts, feelings, and behavioral control can be obtained that they formerly received from alcohol and drugs, we teach them the essence of the 12 steps" (McPeake et al. 1991, pp. 76, 81). Valla and Prince (1989) support this argument when discussing the healing benefits of (ASC-like) religious experiences.

> We have attempted to explore the view that religious experiences are endogenous psychological healing mechanisms analogous to the host of well-known mechanisms for the preservation of bodily homeostasis as described by Cannon and many others.... We have interpreted religious experiences as similar homeostatic mechanisms for the stabilization of self-esteem. We have examined a number of religious experiences as they were reported by an upper-middle-class population during the course of a community survey. Subjects were interviewed about their personal experiences and the life context in which they occurred. In a goodly proportion of cases, these experiences could be interpreted in terms of this self-healing hypothesis. We conclude that the interpretation of religious experiences as self-healing mechanisms does make sense in a high proportion of cases and that the concept is well worth further exploration. [p. 164]

Pigot (1975) makes a similar point:

> What people are doing today is what they have always done. They find, in the midst of material plenty, that they cannot live by bread alone. They seek the beauty, the strangeness of being alive that, despite the coarsening effects of our society, they half perceive to be there on the other side of the veil. They seek it in the only ways that are available to them, by the few remaining avenues left. And one of the remaining avenues is drugs. If we don't like

the picture we see, perhaps we should help each other discover better and more lasting ways of experiencing these aspects of being human, than that of ingesting mind-altering chemicals. [p. 884]

The Native American rehabilitation rituals do attempt precisely that as do most of the other alternative therapies described in this book—reaching for new highs.

6

Therapy through Alternative Achievements: Art Therapy and "Outward Bound" Revitalization

"It is the wounded oyster that mends itself with pearl."
Ralph Waldo Emerson as quoted in Johnson 1990

The problem is not to stop using heroin, the problem is to begin a new life.
Furuholmen 1987

Focus on the Potential!
Greve 1993

Alienation, a sense of meaninglessness, a negative identity perception, and a sense of worthlessness are often proposed as the major reasons people initiate addictive behaviors. In recognition of this, a number of alternative therapies utilize art therapies, other forms of accomplishments (training), as well as stretching addicts' limits through "Outward Bound"–type programs. These are prevalent not only in North America but also in Europe, especially in Scandinavia and France, and probably elsewhere. Such programs, like many of the Native American alternative addict rehabilitation ceremonies, can also be seen as rite-of-passage experiences—a passage to an increased sense of self-worth, sense of accomplishment, and sense of general well-being. Such programs also instill a sense of camaraderie, providing support in various ways, and are similar to the more orthodox therapeutic communities (TCs) in which can be included Alcoholics Anonymous (AA) as well as the harsher (and what some have called the more destructive, rather than particularly therapeutic—although this is debatable) formats such as Synanon, Phoenix House, and Daytop Village.

Some of the U.S. "concept house" TCs have been criticized for treating their patients (inmates?) harshly. Christie and DeBerry (1994) warn that "personnel in therapeutic communities must develop increased sensitivity to the larger cultural factors which influence the construction of the therapeutic community.... Treatment personnel must be careful to avoid constructing therapeutic communities which too closely mirror the larger culture" (p. 803). Yablonsky and Gaylin state, "A true TC does not have a 'we-they' caste system.... The we-they problem does not exist in a true TC structure..." (Yablonsky). Two-tier caste systems can exist in extreme form in concept-house TCs. "The most important thing we face is a rediscovery of community.... We cannot survive without each other. But now, communities have broken down" (Gaylin, cited in Christie and DeBerry 1994, pp. 809–810).

Such harsh programs are particularly prevalent in the United States, while it is claimed that TCs in Britain and elsewhere are more democratic because

> the concept of community... is influenced by the culture within which the community is constructed. It is this influence that we argue undermines the potential effectiveness of the therapeutic community in America.... To conform to an unfair system, one which denies us our individuality,

is to lose some important component of our selves. [Christie and DeBerry 1994, pp. 805, 807]

These authors, and others, argue that although the process in these harsher TCs may resemble the rite-of-passage death-and-rebirth rituals of Native American and other revitalization programs claimed to be therapeutic (successful), the quality of the rebirth, as well as the rapidity of recidivism of the graduates of these programs, raises questions. What is also questioned is the premise of blaming the victim and not considering that there are sociocultural and politico-economic factors that, albeit not to be used as excuses, are significant in the etiology of addictive behavior. Addicts' relative powerlessness within the larger society must be addressed.

> The harsh treatment that drug misusers in TCs receive reflects the original sin view of human development whereby the evil nature of individuals must be eliminated by harsh treatment and punishment. . . . Given the dehumanizing treatment of addicts in TCs, it is not surprising that fewer than 5 to 10% of addicts typically complete such programs. [Christie and DeBerry 1994, p. 814]

Albeit having had some success, it may be that U.S.-based therapeutic communities will not be taken seriously if they make too big a claim about their accomplishments. Peele has suggested,

> "If a drug is consumed in connection with prescribed patterns of behavior and traditional social customs and regulations, it is not likely to cause major problems [coffee, tobacco and, for most, alcohol]. If, on the other hand, either the use or control of the drug is introduced without respect

to existing institutions and cultural practices, and is associated either with political repression or with rebellion, excessive or asocial usage patterns will be present. . . . If it stands for escape and oblivion, then it will be widely misused. This usually happens when a drug is newly introduced to a culture on a large scale [opium in China, alcohol among Native Americans]." [Cited in Christie and DeBerry 1994, p. 812]

Similar to some of the Native American programs, some relatively orthodox (mainstream) addiction programs, as well as purely alternative ones, have included an achievement-oriented challenge segment as part of their overall therapeutic process. For example, the Presbyterian–St. Luke's Medical Center's Addiction Rehabilitation Unit in New York City has established such a therapeutic segment in collaboration with the Colorado Outward Bound School. Such challenges are done within the concept of a TC approach by not only "stretching" the individual but by also showing that success depends on reliance and interaction with others. "The Outward Bound experience has three essential components: a unique physical environment, a unique social environment, and the challenges encountered in learning to cope with both" (Houston and Drum 1990, p. 93). The aims include

> expanding their perceived limits, increasing self esteem and self efficacy, developing interpersonal effectiveness and clarifying their values and spiritual perspectives. . . . Reliance upon others [is] fostered by rigorous outdoor activities, such as rock climbing, hiking, rope crossing, and orienteering. . . .
>
> Outward Bound is a metaphor for real life. . . . The metaphoric experience must be compelling enough to hold the individual's attention. . . . The Outward Bound student does not simply learn or gain insight about his help-related

behavior; rather, the mechanism of the transfer process involves an unconscious connection where the Outward Bound and real life experiences become psychologically identical . . . living two realities simultaneously. . . .

Typically, the group experiences a sense of accomplishment and an awareness that they are not alone and that others are experiencing the same struggle in maintaining their sobriety. . . . The addicts learn to trust and to be trusted. After the group has successfully completed several events, the instructors tend to introduce activities that cause failures or require the addicts to identify and "act out" dysfunctional behavior patterns. [Houston and Drum 1990, pp. 89, 94, 99–100]

Evaluations show that the recidivism rate for those who have participated in this Outward Bound segment is significantly lower than for those who have not.

In Norway and elsewhere in Scandinavia and also in France (Engelmajer 1985) TC therapies often also include such Outward Bound, or wilderness, experiences (Andresen and Waal 1978, Furuholmen 1987, Sandvig 1991, Vaglum 1981). In Norway, there has been a long tradition of using the natural environmental, sports, and the outdoor/mountain life approach to rehabilitation—an example of which is the more than 30-year-old internationally recognized Beitostølen Sportshealth Center working with the disabled (Greve 1993), which has also served as an example for rehabilitation programs working with addicts in Norway and elsewhere. Part of such an outdoor addiction rehabilitation experience involves a camping trip and walking across the Hardangervidda, a high mountain plateau usually inhabited only by reindeer, elk, and the occasional wolf and bear. A sense of individual accomplishment is strengthened as is interdependence with others—the two being complementary rather than contradictory.

There are other ways in which self-confidence and the ability of the detoxified addict can be strengthened, thus minimizing the risk of recidivism. The Skills Training for Adult Recovery (STAR) program in Portland, Oregon is one such alternative that uses a psychoeducational therapeutic process. "A psychoeducational group is a therapeutic experience wherein direct guidance and information about life problems is provided. . . . [It is] aimed at improving day-to-day problem solving and coping skills techniques in the treatment of addiction disorders" (LaSalvia 1993, pp. 441, 443).

A special psychoeducational program includes the use of music intervention, primarily to stimulate memory and to reinforce psychoeducational messages. Other alternatives include occupational therapy in addict rehabilitation programs (Stensrud and Lushbough 1988).

Art therapy, especially when patients are part of a group, can be particularly important in the rehabilitation process. "This positive support of the group at her revelation of her negative traits [through the reading of her poetry] is a crucial part of the healing ritual. . . . What intrigues me the most about art therapy is how insightful patients are about each other's [artistic expressions]" (Johnson 1990, p. 302). The members of an art therapy group, conceived as a therapeutic community, also constitute an alternative rehabilitation process that is able to strengthen the participants' sense of self-worth, capabilities, and positive identities.

Johnson (1990) has come to realize that a major issue in rehabilitation is the problem of shame:

> Shame about our failures and imperfections and rejections began at such an early age that most of us are unaware that underlying our present suffering is a belief that there is something basically wrong with us. Shame becomes our

identity, and once "shame is transformed into an identity it becomes toxic and dehumanizing" (Bradshaw). . . . Surrounding this hidden belief in a flawed self is terrible pain and fear of being exposed. [p. 301]

Johnson uses drama and poetry to work with patients in a "shamanic" therapeutic way (in that she considers herself as a "wounded healer"—as all of us are wounded—who has healed her own "wound") through poetry and drama: "Listening to and the creation of poetry are important acts of self-healing. . . . Robert Graves wrote that his poetry is 'the record of my individual struggle from darkness towards some measure of light'" (p. 301), and thus similarly and empathetically she develops a therapeutic bond with her patients.

> In drama and dance therapy, it is possible to achieve group catharsis through the spontaneous creation of an imaginary domain in which everyone participates and has a role. . . . Laughter and playfulness are essential for healing as "a sense of humor may be the ultimate criteria for measuring a person's recovery from internalized shame" (Bradshaw). . . . We write a poem, we draw a picture, we act in a play, and we come a little closer to understanding ourselves, to forgiving ourselves, to healing ourselves. Creativity is an antidote to shame, connecting us with our Creator-Higher Power, and our true Selves, allowing us to turn liabilities into assets, wounds into pearls. [pp. 303, 306–307]

Another art therapist, using creative writing, presents the relevance of this approach as follows:

> When the youths were asked direct questions related to how they felt, most became defensive or drew a blank because they could not identify how they felt. By using sight,

sound, texture, taste, smell, feeling and shape to elicit emotional responses, feelings became more understandable and less threatening to the youths. [McDonald 1985, p. 130]

Others use so-called bibliotherapy by which key reading materials, including books, are read and discussed and often serve as an introduction to the participation in successful therapeutic sessions, since the patients have been "opened up" by the reading material discussed (Pardeck 1991). Mahony and Waller (1992, pp. 176–177) also discuss art therapy as a means of "breaking down resistance to treatment [because] art can provide a safe form of expression that allows the addict a glimpse of his authentic self."

Both the artistically creative and the Outward Bound "stretching" approaches (reaching new highs) aim at placing the patient in touch with the authentic self and restoring the patient's sense of positive identity, a sense of worth, as well as a sense of community and an ability to cope. He can contemplate an accomplishment and can say, "I can do this! I am able!" and through this reduce alienation and isolation. These methods may be important because they do all of this—especially bringing about a sense of satisfaction, and, significantly, an increased affect—but such Outward Bound and artistic activities may also stimulate the endorphins and be therapeutically effective because of the positive effect resulting from being able to bring about natural highs.

7

Biofeedback and Religious, Spiritual, and Meditation Therapies

> The programme's not a rehabilitation programme per se but is a means of self-development.
> Clements et al. 1988

> Was not their excessive use of alcohol in itself a perverted form of search for some measure of enlightenment or higher consciousness!?
> Buxton et al. 1987

> Getting high is the rite of passage to another world or another, preferred, state of mind.
> Roman 1977

Biofeedback

Biofeedback and general relaxation techniques have been used since the 1970s to assist in addiction therapy as a substitute for opiates and in enabling patients to stimulate endogenous "highs" (stimulating endorphins). "Reports indicate that sensations of well being and *pleasure* [emphasis added] accompany this process" (Lamontagne et al. 1975, p. 337). It also enables patients to have insight into their own destructive and constructive behavior and to make "the client more aware of the therapeutic issues he had to work on in order to stabilize his life" (Brinkman 1978, p. 823). That biofeedback is used successfully by nonaddicted patients to reduce anxiety and for a number of health problems, including gastric ulcers, insomnia, high blood pressure, to mention but a few (Brown 1975), may also serve to prevent future addictive behavior.

Since one reason for taking drugs is thought to be due to states of high tension and anxiety, biofeedback, to reduce anxiety, has been shown to be effective both as a preventive and as a therapeutic measure. While recognizing the relevance of relaxation techniques in addiction therapy, Klajner and colleagues (1984) believe that it is not so much the reduction in anxiety that is the crucial factor, although this is important, but rather the increased control obtained (and perceived to be obtained) by the patient.

Roszell and Chaney (1982) are more cautious than others but state that "although autogenic training is no panacea, it is a useful modality in the drug abuse treatment armamentarium" (p. 1337). One problem noted with this therapeutic modality, however, was the difficulty in getting patients to practice relaxation feedback techniques once some restoration of a normal life had been achieved.

A recent study by Denne and colleagues (1991) has confirmed the results reported in the 1970s and 1980s (Brinkman 1978, Roszell and Chaney 1982):

> The effect of the amount of biofeedback training received upon abstinence from alcohol was studied at 3, 6 and 12 months post-discharge for 233 male veterans in an inpatient alcoholic rehabilitation unit. The frequency of sobriety for those patients with at least 6 training sessions was significantly better than for those with less or no training at all three time periods. [p. 335]

Meditation

Meditation (including both meditative and physical yoga) practices have long been seen as efficacious alternative therapies for addiction. Much has been written about the role of a special form of meditation practice, transcendental meditation (TM), in this regard.

One of the best known early articles on TM and addiction was that by Benson and Wallace (1972) based on a study of 1,862 subjects, which indicated a marked reduction in drug use and also in tobacco and alcohol consumption by meditators. They speculated that one of the reasons for this was the physiological changes brought about by meditation.

> During TM oxygen consumption and heart rate significantly decrease, skin resistance significantly increases, and the electroencephalogram shows predominantly slow alpha wave activity with occasional theta wave activity. Thus, the practice of TM is physiologically distinguished from sitting quietly with eyes open or closed, from sleeping or dreaming, and from the relaxation or rest suggested by hypnosis. [p. 374]

A more recent review, noting 350 research studies on TM in twenty-five countries, confirms TM's relevance for addiction rehabilitation and particularly as a means of preventing addiction (Clements et al. 1988). Interestingly, the authors make the same point made by a number of others working with different addiction rehabilitation programs, namely that, "the programme is not a rehabilitation programme per se, but is a means of self-development" (p. 51).

In another, more recent, careful review of twenty-four TM and addiction studies, Gelderloos and colleagues (1991) not only report that all twenty-four studies showed the positive effect of TM but, again, linked TM with more fundamental developmental issues:

> It is easier to eliminate substance dependence by providing an alternative gratifying experience, especially one having positive long-term effects. . . . It is an ongoing engagement to attain higher levels of psychological integration and health. . . . During TM [practitioners attain] an experience of inner contentment or bliss, . . . feelings of happiness, contentment and fulfillment [as well as] positive affect. [pp. 294, 296, 313]

They also point out that "even the successful 12 step Alcoholics Anonymous program includes a 'spiritual development' component" (p. 295).

But, as with biofeedback and most of the other alternative methods reported on here, Gelderloos and colleagues point out that the efficacy may also be seen as linked to biochemical-produced changes.

> TM increases the effectiveness of melatonin in preventing or eliminating stress. Increase in the effectiveness of systems such as the serotonin and melatonin systems which mediate important coping mechanisms is consistent with the ability of TM to reduce and prevent substance misuse. . . . Neurochemicals and neuroendocrine research appears to be uncovering plausible mechanisms by which TM could produce both short and long term benefits in the treatment of drug use. . . .
>
> TM provides a natural way to achieve the experience substance users are looking for: relief from distress, increased self-esteem, enhancement of well-being and self-efficacy, and a sense of personal power and meaning in life. . . .

> One result is an enhanced sensitivity to the negative influence of foreign substances. This increased sensitivity could be responsible for the sudden "distaste" for drugs reported by many who learn TM. . . .
> Neuroendocrine systems, being a link between the basic biochemical processes of the cell and the overall psychological state of the organism, may be one of the most fruitful areas for the further exploration of these mechanisms. [pp. 317–318]

Others, such as Ganguli (1985), also suggest not only that efficacy may depend on the mediative practices themselves (nor only with the associated biochemical changes), but also

> that membership of these meditation groups or subcultures serves the same or allied psychological needs as drugs do and therefore the meditation-centered activities of such groups serve as a substitute for drug use. . . . Stanley Einstein has said: "The greater the involvement with drugs, the less the involvement with people." The reverse also seems to be true. [pp. 960–961]

TM for addiction rehabilitation has also received negative reviews. An early study by Anderson (1977) for one, concluded, on the basis of a study of eighty-nine subjects, that "TM cannot be offered to any group of drug abusers with the expectation that they will turn away from their drugs and embrace meditation" (p. 1309), the suggestion being that the method can only be successful for certain (self-) selected groups of addicts already positively disposed to meditation.

Galanter and Buckley (1978) suggest that meditative practices other than TM can also be effective; they report on the practices of the Divine Light Mission (DLM) established in the United States in 1971:

> Quantitative studies on the clinical effects of meditation have until now been restricted to transcendental meditation. Clinical findings have been reported with regard to general psychiatric symptoms and for diminution in alcohol and marijuana use. . . . The intensity of transcendental experiences reported during meditation (DLM) is striking, and each of these experiences served as a predictor for decline of one or more of the symptoms. [p. 691]

A psychological rather than biological form of feedback, *psychodrama*, has also been used with some success in treating addicts in different parts of the world (Crawford 1989, Dushman and Bressler 1991).

Spiritualism

As already noted, the relevance of a spiritual approach to addiction rehabilitation is not just one that can be associated with so-called esoteric spiritualist sects; it is much more profound than a simplistic reading of the Marxist dictum that "religion is the opiate of the people." We should also be careful not to equate spirituality with religion because they are different (Buxton et al. 1987). Spirituality, or the importance of spiritual development, is central to the twelve-step rehabilitative approach of such a mainstream therapeutic program as Alcoholics Anonymous, step two of which suggests that healing depends on coming to "believe that a Power greater than ourselves could restore us to sanity" (Buxton et al. 1987, p. 280). Smith (1994, p. 111) recently quoted Jung to support the importance of spirituality in the AA approach: "Jung: 'the compulsion to use alcohol is so great that it is likely that only a spiritual experience could overwhelm that compulsion.'"

Although the distinction between spirituality and religion should be recognized, it is clear from the previous sections that religion and religious teachings are central to many successful alternative addiction therapeutic programs throughout the world. However, unlike other findings, a study by Zucker and colleagues (1987) showed that degree of religiosity among patients in a Veterans Administration (VA) medical center alcohol treatment center was not a significant factor in the personal histories of alcohol use. They conclude, rather, that "it could be postulated that the conflict between religious teachings and the compulsion to drink in religious alcoholics is an important source of increases stress and anxiety" (p. 52).

Considering spiritualism slightly differently, it is clear that a number of Latino spiritualists and black spiritual churches effectively rehabilitate alcoholics in the United States. Many Latinos, for example, find the mainstream rehabilitation programs alien and do not use them. Singer and Borrero (1984) describe the use of a spiritual center by Puerto Rican alcoholics and their families and friends in Hartford, Connecticut, among whom alcoholism is conceptualized as caused by the invasion of one or more evil spirits, with the central aspect of therapy thus being to discover the identity of the spirit so that it can be expelled and sometimes replaced by a benevolent spirit.

This is a process performed by a center's medium and usually involves attempting to "pass" the harmful spirit from the client so that it will possess the medium (healer) instead. In this way the medium can identify and communicate with it, and thus appease it. "Passing" a spirit is considered a life-threatening act. The therapeutic process of getting rid of the evil spirit contains a number of ritualistic steps that also involve family and friends as well as the alcoholic client and the healer.

> Special candles and incense from the botanica are burned in the alcoholic's home to give the offending spirit "light" and raise it from its confused and liminal state.

Finally, a friend or relative is requested to bring a bottle of liquor to be "fixed" by the mediums: . . . let this person get sick when he drinks this liquor. Every time he drinks, let him get sick. [The healers] . . . actively involve the concerned friends and relatives of the drinker in culturally meaningful acts of homeopathic and contagious magic.

Friends and relatives are able to feel that they are working to heal the drinker, and the resulting change in *their* [my emphasis] attitude may indeed contribute to this end. . . .

There are a number of concrete acts for the clients to perform, acts which are structured, repetitive, and tied to an orderly development. Directed spiritual treatment appears to offer a regulated life-style for alcoholic clients [Singer and Borrero 1984, pp. 259–60, 262]

Clients are also instructed to take special baths at home, to say special prayers and "to light candles and make offerings to the saints . . . to cleanse their homes of malevolent forces. . . . The mediums provide a special cleansing in the back room of the centro. This involved rubbing spiritual oils on the drinker's stomach. . . . The mediums also prescribe several herbal teas, including anise, peppermint, and garlic to be consumed three times a week in various combinations" (Singer and Borrero 1984, p. 261).

This form of therapy does not function on the spiritual plane alone nor does it focus on the patient alone, since such therapies also deal with mundane, material matters, such as solving interpersonal conflicts, employment problems, and the like. The healers work in many ways as family therapists and they focus on "rebuilding family relations and channels of communication, mobilizing the family as a supportive network, shielding the alcoholic from familiar drinking contexts, and involving the family in the therapeutic community offered by the centro" (p. 265). In addition to helping the patient to face his problems and to deal with them, the healers concentrate on the special significance that dignity and respect (*dignidad y respeto*) as well as the "mother" have for Puerto Ricans and Latinos in general, to a greater extent than for other Americans. Stopping alcohol abuse will be a way to regain *dignidad* and *respeto* and to please one's mother. "Puerto Ricans reported 1) sadness, crying, desperation in relation to actual or potential loss of their mother, 2) positive feelings about themselves as a result of their relationship with their mother, and 3) the need to follow their mother's dictates" (p. 262).

Singer and Borrero conclude by confirming that

> folk treatment is culturally appropriate not only because it employs culturally valued symbols, roles, and relationships, but because it mobilizes them in light of the ever-changing context of group life and experiences....
>
> Indigenous treatment... has its own shortcomings... and offers no panacea for contemporary global alcohol crisis.... But folk treatment does incorporate insights and strategies more closely aligned with the special needs, meaning systems, and changing experience of so-called special populations, and hence may hold important lessons for new directions in alcohol treatment. [p. 269]

Baer (1981), for one, reports the use of medium therapists (or spiritual advisors or prophets) for patients/adherents of black spiritual churches in the United States.

> Most individuals who seek Spiritual advisors have "conditions" rather than ailments... financial and domestic difficulties... a son who repeatedly runs into trouble with the law or who is on drugs... alcoholism.... Black Spiritual religion with its complex of prophets and advisors provides

people with a theology for existence and survival. . . . It . . . is a "practical and utilitarian religion which cares more for earthly than heavenly goings-on" in that it emphasizes the acquisition of health, love, economic prosperity, and interpersonal power. [pp. 155, 163]

While the spiritual advisors and the general participation in these churches "enable clients, at least to some extent, to overcome a state of 'demoralization,' . . . they have lost confidence in their abilities to cope with the pressures of everyday problems" (p. 164).

Baer suggests that there is a tendency here to "blame the victim" (in a different way from the Latino spiritist centers, which also address contextual issues) and to overlook the socioeconomic and political context within which black addicts live their lives, and the significance of this context in the etiology and maintenance of addiction. He concludes by suggesting that, albeit helpful, "the message that 'therapy can solve everything' . . . may serve to frustrate those undergoing treatment even more once they come to the realization that this cannot be the case. . . . While the Spiritual religion and its complex of mediums appears to provide an important coping mechanism for a segment of the Black community, at best it tends to be ameliorative" (p. 166).

In addition to AA and the previously mentioned spiritual therapeutic alternatives, Christian Science (CS) is another alternative addiction therapy modality. CS holds that "all misfortune, including disease, is . . . viewed as a mistaken belief in the existence of a material reality separate from God. . . . Sickness is a dream from which the patient needs to be awakened. . . . Healing involves the realization that it is impossible to be sick" (Singer 1982, p. 3).

While CS "therapists" do recognize that people get drunk,

they deny the ability of alcohol itself to cause intoxication and to have chemical or behavioral consequences, since drunkenness is caused not by the alcohol but rather by the alcoholic's belief and expectations. Thus therapy lies in changing individuals' beliefs and expectations. "Treatment of alcoholism in CS involves a 'ritualistically repeated denial' of these underlying psychological problems and the urge to drink, combined with an equally ritualized 'acceptance of oneself as the loved child of God.' ... The practitioners focused on the patient's emotional state while denying the reality of their problems" (pp. 5–6).

CS therapy differs from an AA approach, both in that it rejects the reality of alcoholism as most of us understand it and in that it aims at creating an individual who should be "a self-governing human being with strong inner convictions and controls" (p. 9)—it is a willpower model of therapy.

Being, similar to Baer, a critical medical anthropologist concerned with the importance of a "political-economy of health" perspective, Singer concludes,

> All individually oriented alcoholism therapies are limited in that they focus on treatment rather than prevention. So long as enormous social structural contradictions and stresses prevail, so long as social problems like alcoholism are privatized as individual problems, and so long as alcohol consumption is profitably promoted as a recreational outlet, the scale of the current alcoholism problem is not likely to diminish. [p. 11]

Ritual

As was seen to be a major aspect of some Native American therapies, a number of other alternative addiction rehabilitation programs focus on the importance of the therapeutic effects of ritual, in and of itself.

> The project... would offer its participants a place and time in which they could change their state of being, through symbolic actions, and so to "kill" their inadequate "addict-part" in a ritualistic ceremony of Tchia, rebirth and resurrection. This will be followed by a peak ceremony of renewing self-awareness in which the initiated will seek and earn permission to live his new "clean" life.... The individuals will be taught a replacement ritual, ie. something to be taken home and performed every day, in order to reinforce the new positive, clean life style. [They are] encouraged to form a new identity to replace the negative junkie image. [Roman 1977, p. 352]

DeRios and Smith (1977), among others, point out that drug use has been pervasive within most cultures in the world, and especially so in the Americas, but the very ritualistic (and often sacred) format within which drugs were used acted as a control measure against addiction (Furst 1972). Healing (including shamanic) rituals also include the use of hallucinogenic drugs, but, because of the ritualistic and controlled circumstances, they have therapeutic rather than addictive consequences (Emboden and DeRios 1981, Prince 1988, Ripinsky-Naxon 1989, Tiwari et al. 1990).

> Fear, rage, despair, disorganization, and other intense emotions result when an individual's identity is threatened. ... A salvation ritual may enable the victim to regain his sense of worth . . . [such as the] Peyote [ritual] by many American Indian populations... [or] a West African revitalization or nativistic movement called the Bwiti Cult, where the hallucinogenic plant Tabernanthe Iboga is used by the Fang people to ameliorate the effects of a century of French colonial policy. [DeRios and Smith 1977, p. 270]

However, DeRios and Smith do recognize that drug use rituals can be both negative and positive, especially when played out in contemporary North American and European contexts. "[There are] several types of ritual. One is ritual as therapy and anti-therapy. . . . The ritual is intended to control human health for therapeutic or anti-therapeutic purposes. . . . 'Ritual of rebellion' . . . use of heroin, stimulants and psychedelics may be a way in which such rebellion is manifested" (pp. 270–271).

Nevertheless, DeRios and Smith maintain that learning the ritual and the ritualistic use of drugs itself is a way to inhibit addiction and to limit the destructive (and potentially heighten the positive) aspects of drug taking.

> In contemporary American society, then, group development of appropriate rituals and social sanctions, has led to a diminution of problems of a psychological or physiological nature associated with drug use. . . .
> Adolescents and young adults with considerable experience with marijuana rituals may have trouble managing the use of alcohol because they are, in effect, unfamiliar with the rituals that provide a means to control that drug's effects. . . .
> Australian aboriginal populations who in prehistoric times used a scopolamine containing plant, pituri, within a ritualized pattern began to have rampant problems with alcohol once that drug was introduced to them. [pp. 273–274]

This is the argument also used by Zinberg and colleagues (1975), who suggest that addiction can be drastically reduced through sanctioned but controlled and ritualistic use of drugs by those so inclined. They base their argument on the fact that though alcoholism is a serious problem, most alcohol use is nonaddicted and done within certain socially (ritualistically) sanctioned and familiar patterns. "Alcohol has the potential for psychological and physiological harm as great as any drug known, but the vast majority of its users manage relatively controlled use" (Zinberg et al. 1975, p. 176). In a study of nonaddicted drug users, they suggest that a major reason preventing addiction among this group of drug users was the controlled and ritualistic manner in which drugs were used: "To our surprise, sanctions and rituals, despite their underground existence, were operating more successfully in the direction of preventing abuse than the larger culture had a right to expect" (p. 174).

Because of the illegality of the drugs, however, they were used in a covert manner, associated with potentially negative consequences. Zinberg and colleagues used the results of their study to argue for the legalization but controlled and ritualistic use of drugs, which they felt would drastically reduce both the criminality and the addictive behavior associated with current drug use.

8

Acupuncture Therapies

> There are clinical investigations into detoxification by [acupuncture] electro stimulation where electro stimulation has been shown to be effective. . . . These benefits—rapid and substantial reduction of the acute withdrawal syndrome; significant amelioration of the chronic withdrawal syndrome; and minimal psychic distress and aggression during treatment—assessed and measured by a variety of physiological and psychological criteria—prove to be significantly detailed and predictable, regardless of the chemical of addiction being treated, or country or facility in which the investigation took place.
>
> Patterson et al. 1993

The seeming effectiveness of acupuncture in easing withdrawal pains was accidentally discovered in Hong Kong in 1972 and reported by Wen and Cheung (1973). One of the patients Wen treated in 1972 for a lung problem turned out also to have been an opium addict, who despite an inability to satisfy his (addict) habit while spending an extensive period in hospital, did not experience withdrawal symptoms. Acupuncture and electrical stimulation specifically use the lung (and heart) points in the left ear. With repeated stimulation addicts are reported to be relieved of withdrawal symptoms in a matter of days. Subsequently, a patient may receive additional stimulation treatments whenever he feels a craving for drugs.

After discovering its relevance for addiction therapy, Wen continued treating addicts with acupuncture in Hong Kong, and

Kao and Lu (1974) also reported on their efforts there. Acupuncture is now extensively used in various countries in Southeast Asia, in Australia, in the United States, and in Europe, in the treatment of opiate and other drug addicts as well as alcoholics (Equinox Group 1988, Lau 1976, Newmeyer et al. 1984, Sainsbury 1974, M. O. Smith 1988a,b, Smith and Khan 1988). In 1993 "approximately 200 clinics, in 32 states [in the U.S.] offer[ed] auricular acupuncture for the treatment [of cocaine and other drug addiction]" (Margolin et al. 1993, p. 103). It should be noted that acupuncture treatment is now no longer considered an exotic or "fringe" therapeutic choice, which some called, for example, the Haight-Ashbury Free Medical Clinic, which was one of the first places in the U.S. to use acupuncture in the treatment of addicts (albeit, initially, with mixed results because of its "foreignness") (Newmeyer and Whitehead 1977, Newmeyer et al. 1984).

Since 1974,

> Lincoln Hospital, New York City, has used acupuncture as the primary method of treatment for drug-addicted persons. Acupuncture relieves withdrawal symptoms, prevents the craving for drugs and increases the rate of participation of patients in long-term treatment programmes. The best results have been obtained by treating patients in an open-group setting, using acupuncture points in the external ear with needles without electrical stimulation. The same points are used at each visit, regardless of the type of drug to which the person is addicted. [Smith and Khan 1988, p. 35]

Patterson (1974, 1975), who first worked with Dr. Wen in Hong Kong, subsequently set up an acupuncture addiction treatment center in England and later carried the method to the

United States. She has written extensively about its efficacy in addiction treatment (Patterson 1993, Patterson et al. 1993). She is now convinced that

> [it is] not the acupuncture system which produced these clinical effects, but the type of electrical signal which we used transcranially. . . . I have named my treatment Neuro-Electric Therapy (NET). . . . The precise techniques of the successful application of NET include the exact siting of the electrodes, above the mastoid process, and the polarity of the electrodes. . . . Most crucial of all is the delivery of the correct—and highly precise—pulse frequency. [Patterson 1993, p. 1]

In another article she and her colleagues similarly assert that "the specific parameters of electrical current application were central to therapeutic success" (Patterson et al. 1993, p. 131).

She also casts some doubt about the value of acupuncture "to produce *rapid* [my emphasis] detoxification" if it is not combined with electrostimulation: "There is no published evidence that acupuncture, without potentiation of this very weak current by electric stimulation of appropriate parameters, can produce a rapid detoxification from any addictive drugs" (Patterson et al. 1993, p. 138).

Later studies have affirmed both its efficacy as a therapeutic modality, and many are in agreement about the mechanisms responsible for its success (Brumbaught 1993, Bullock et al. 1989, Margolin et al. 1993, Patterson 1993, Patterson et al. 1993, Smith and Khan 1988, Wen 1980, Yang and Kwok 1986). Others, while willing to admit that acupuncture may be helpful for certain individuals, are more skeptical (i.e., Whitehead 1978).

More than a decade after Whitehead's study, Riet and colleagues (1990, p. 379) carried out a similar review of "22 controlled clinical studies on the efficacy of acupuncture in three fields of addiction: cigarette smoking (15), heroin (5), and alcohol (2)," and concluded that, "controlled clinical research on acupuncture and addiction is scarce, although the results of a controlled clinical trial on addiction to alcohol have recently been published." The study of which they approved was the one reported by Bullock and colleagues (1989), which claimed the efficacy of acupuncture in treating alcoholics: "Our findings show that acupuncture can be effective for treatment of severe recidivist alcoholics" (p. 1438). They added that "increased use of acupuncture therapy may eventually lead to a decrease in the number of inpatient admissions to expensive treatment centers" (p. 1438). This point is also being made by a number of others (e.g., Smith and Khan 1988). M. O. Smith (1988a) reports:

> Dr. Bernard Bihari, the Director of Kings County, reports that psychotic cocaine users who used to have to be hospitalized are now routinely treated on an out-patient basis with acupuncture and individual counseling. . . .
> We would never claim that acupunture alone is an adequate treatment for crack abuse. . . . Nevertheless acupuncture detoxification with counseling seems to be an adequate means of reaching the early sobriety stage of treatment for today's cocaine abusers. . . . Acupuncture detoxification is then a popular, inexpensive foundation for successful outpatient and self-help modalities. [p. 246]

Yet, a report on a meeting at the National Institute for Drug Abuse (NIDA) "by a panel of experts in the field of substance abuse treatment research" decided that "the consensus was that much fundamental work remains to be done and that after two decades of contemporary use in the field of addiction treatment, there is no compelling evidence for the efficacy of acupuncture in the treatment of either opiate or cocaine dependence" (McLelland et al. 1993, p. 575).

A small study of alcoholics carried out by Worner and colleagues (1992) also found no grounds to support the claim that acupuncture was therapeutically efficacious and "caution-[ed] against the routine use of this treatment" (p. 169).

While it is fairly well established that acupuncture is effective in providing significant relief to patients during detoxification, it is less certain whether it contributes to greater long-term abstinence rates than other therapies. Early reports were careful to distinguish between detoxification treatment and rehabilitation and to make disclaimers about the tenacity of abstinence through use of this method (Kao and Lu 1974). As noted above, a number of articles point to the value of acupuncture, but many take pains in adding that long-term efficacy can only be achieved in concert with, and as a way to make the patient ready for, psychological and other counseling therapies that can expect to have a longer lasting effect (Brumbaugh 1993, Schuckit 1993, M. O. Smith 1988a, Washburn et al. 1993).

Schuckit (1993, p. 3) stated that "acupuncture is likely to be of optimal use only when combined with additional treatment such as counseling, education, outreach to the family." According to Smith and Khan (1988), "Acupuncture detoxification is a non-judgmental, nurturing process. It blends well with most crisis counselling and long term rehabilitation programmes." Patterson (1993, p. 3) also confirms that "psychotherapy and support systems remain an important part of the treatment." In an earlier work she stated (also see Chapter 7):

> Another outstanding feature of this type of therapy is that, in addition to having his physical symptoms eased, the addict becomes immediately responsive to behavioral therapy. . . .

> More and more patients are crowding our clinics with the complaint of an inner emptiness, the sense of a total and utter meaninglessness of life. . . . Any possible form of therapy for drug addiction, caused to a great extent by the lack of this "will to meaning" in the lives of the sufferers, must also take into consideration at an early stage the communication of a new set of spiritual values. . . . [We must treat] spiritually as well as medically. [Patterson 1975, pp. 66, 82]

Many feel that the evaluations of acupuncture programs are still not substantial enough to warrant a definitive statement on the method. Yet others, such as Patterson and Smith, for example, are strongly convinced of the efficacy of this method. Smith and Khan (1988) conclude:

> Research carried out at the University of Minnesota and the Downstate Medical Center in the U.S. have confirmed that acupuncture substantially reduces withdrawal symptoms and the craving for drugs. . . . Positive results have been obtained using acupuncture detoxification of patients dependent on cocaine, opiates, phencyclidine or alcohol. [p. 36]

9

Salient Features of Alternative Therapies and Implications for Future Addiction Programs

> It must be hoped that in the future there will be much more open exchange of ideas than has sometimes been seen, with no one dominant cultural view. This is a vital consideration equally for treatment, preventive action and research. Drugs are again only the exemplar of wider problems, and at worst of the general belief that if foreigners are not like us, they are wrong.
>
> To listen to other countries' experiences, one must first be given a chance to hear of those experiences. In relation to drugs, an enormous amount is being thought about, argued about, and accomplished in many different countries, and further ways of exchanging these experiences are badly needed.
>
> Edwards and Arif 1983

There are a number of similar features in the different alternative therapies practiced throughout the world. These may be considered in relation to detoxification on the one hand and activities that support abstinence on the other, although many activities are not so clearly delineated; for example, activities that primarily facilitate detoxification may also have long-term rehabilitative effects on abstinence, and activities primarily concerned with abstinence and the revitalization of the patient may contribute to biochemical changes that are effective during detoxification and in inhibiting withdrawal symptoms.

Albeit some therapies focus more on detoxification than on long-term rehabilitation, almost all alternative approaches are concerned with both of these aspects of addiction therapy. Rehabilitation, in terms of long-term abstinence of an addict who can maintain and live a fulfilled life without addiction, is the ultimate test of any therapy, yet all therapies must first deal with the immediacy of detoxification. Several alternative approaches use herbal mixtures to facilitate detoxification since these are said to reduce withdrawal pain and the craving for drugs. Similarly, acupuncture (and electrostimulation) is also primarily a means for facilitating detoxification, although it can also be used subsequently on a continuing basis to lessen the craving for drugs. Physical stimulation through repeated and rhythmic chanting, physical exertion, dancing, and even meditation is used in detoxification. These methods are seen to affect the endorphins and to cause biochemical changes in the body that trigger the opiate receptor and produce a so-called endogenous, or internal, "high," minimizing the need for external stimulants. Some argue that the pain of "cold turkey" withdrawal is a necessary shock, the traumatic experience of which will prevent anyone who has gone through it from returning to drug use. However, most alternative practitioners would argue that no therapy can begin to be successful without stimulating the endorphins or effecting biochemical changes.

Many of the activities used for physical stimulation during detoxification can also be practiced regularly over time for continued maintenance of a drug-free state. Acupuncture and electrostimulation (facilitated by the invention of a portable stimulator and other equipment that can be used at home) have already been mentioned; the repeated but controlled use of peyote is another, as is regular physical exercise such as running or dancing, all of which are said to produce endogenous "highs," approaching that obtained by use of exogenous hallucinogenic stimulants. But other, less mechanistic, features that are not primarily characterized by repeated physical stimulation are also common to many of these therapeutic approaches and appear significant in the maintenance of abstinence over time.

We may theorize that many of these are linked to etiological perceptions of addiction. For example, and as mentioned in the first chapter, alienation, identity crisis, or repeated negative identity feedback—often as a result of racism or poverty—can be linked to the fairly universal alternative therapeutic attempts at revitalization, the creation of a positive identity, and mobilizing processes that will bring the former addict from a state of despair and meaninglessness to one of positive self-esteem and meaningful engagement, in which he is imbued with energy. Many programs, including the orthodox Alcoholics Anonymous, emphasize the importance of developing the addict's spiritual side (often quite distinct from adherence to formal religious groups). Because of this, many of the therapies discussed can be seen, and often see themselves, as transformative events, the main purpose of which is the transformation of the former addict into a renewed and positive self. Whether some conceptualize the therapeutic process in terms of the performance of rites of passage or of death and rebirth revitalization rituals, what is shared is a conviction that for addiction therapy to have a lasting effect requires what, for the lack of a better term, may be called fostering and nurturing human development.

But as addiction is not necessarily, or primarily, the result of personality disorders, blaming the victim or focusing, in a medicalized way, on an addict's possible biochemical pathology can be destructive and antitherapeutic and is at least scientifically ambiguous, if not of insignificant scientific merit. Such human development must include coping mechanisms for facing the everyday world from which escape is difficult and which provides fertile ground for the temptations of drug abuse. Eventually the addict is back in the world, back in his old neighborhood, and many of the alternative therapeutic processes are dedicated to help him to function differently than before. Thus, although some of us may be convinced that a major factor in reducing addiction depends first on demand reduction—and not primarily on supply reduction (that will follow)—which in turn is related to, and requires, social therapy, social transformation, and a fight against sociopolitical and ethnic inequity and discrimination (created by the making of the "inferior other"), a first step becomes the transformation and empowerment of individual addicts. Some programs accomplish this by recognizing social causative factors, without considering the individual addict a victim, but rather someone who needs to take responsibility for his own life. Incorporating this perception and using it to guide rehabilitation is precisely what is basic to many alternative addiction therapies.

A positive self-image and a sense of power over one's life—power in facing and shaping the circumstances of one's life—are what most therapeutic programs attempt to create, but linked to this many also recognize the apparent innate desire of all human beings to periodically achieve altered states of consciousness—to be ecstatic, euphoric, awed, or elated—to be "high." Some find such "highs" through spirituality and meditation, others through creative endeavors, and yet others through walks in nature, white-water rafting, mountaineering, or through doing "good deeds" (Dharma); there are many possibilities. Others seek such euphoria and escape from everyday realities through alcohol and drugs. Many of the therapies discussed here recognize this innate need to achieve "highs" and part of the therapeutic process is showing the addicts that these can be reached by nondestructive means. Even when drugs are used, such as the regular ingestion of peyote by members of the Native American Church, this is done in a ritualistic and controlled, nonaddictive manner in which fellowship and spiritual connectedness are the most important features.

Through the two-step (but usually integrated) process of immediate detoxification and rehabilitation for long-term abstinence, most alternative therapies engage addicts in a process of transformation and revitalization—often taking the form of a death and rebirth ritual—by which a positive self-image is created and a sense of power is instilled, including coping mechanisms for facing an unchanged everyday world, and through which the addicts realize that different and more profound "highs" can be achieved without reliance on drugs.

Implications for Future Addiction Programs

One of the basic lessons of alternative therapies confirms what is also realized by a review of orthodox methods—that successful detoxification, no matter how ably it is carried out, is but a small, albeit significant, initial step of a comprehensive and lasting addiction therapy. Repeated use of acupuncture or electrostimulations, as well as the continued use of herbal and other substances (such as methadone, although many claim its use merely substitutes one addictive substance for another) can reduce an addict's cravings and help maintain abstinence. The relative efficacy of such long-term maintenance mechanisms does confirm the importance of a concern for biomedical processes and physiological yearnings. However, one must distinguish between drug-free maintenance through repeated interventions and comprehensive therapy, even though such therapy may also encourage the former addict to engage in new activities on a regular basis.

It is important to distinguish between maintenance and therapy out of a concern for the negative psychosocial and spiritual antecedents and aspects of addiction, not only its physical attributes. Once again, the concern is with alienation, identity crisis, or negative identity perception (and feedback) and a sense of meaninglessness and hopelessness. The use of drugs is both a search for ecstasy and an escape from an unacceptable, stressful, or repugnant reality (is it ever only for "kicks"?). Thus, the more important lessons to be learned from alternative therapeutic approaches are the attention to transformation, to revitalization, to human [and spiritual] development, and to the search for happiness and euphoria. Within this context, the measure of success can only start, but not be satisfied, with abstinence (maintenance of a drug-free state) since comprehensive therapy should also lead a former addict to regain a positive self-image, to have a sense of power over the circumstances of his life (beyond merely coping within the same negative environment from which he came), to begin to fulfill his human potentials, possibly including enhanced creativity and spirituality, and to have a sense of well-being and the potential for euphoric experiences.

Therapy must consider the sociocultural, economic, and political environment to which the former addict will likely return and provide him with practical, psychological, and spiritual means to survive and to thrive following therapy. This is a tall order. Yet, such comprehensiveness is something most alternative therapies attempt to approximate, and it is a focus that should at least be attempted by all addiction therapy programs. The formation of a support-group network may be the follow-up to therapy, as might be the regular, and even ritual, interaction with members of such a support community. Other consequences include engagement in new activities, including meditation or artistic pursuits. The pursuit of such practices should allow for the possibility to stimulate endogenous "highs" and to achieve euphoria and an afterglow of well-being—to reach new highs.

PART II
Annotated Bibliography

1
Acupuncture

Brumbaugh, A. G. (1993). Acupuncture: new perspectives in chemical dependency treatment. *Journal of Substance Abuse Treatment* 10:35–43.

Bullock, M. L., Culliton, P. D., and Olander, R. T. (1989). Controlled trial of acupuncture for severe recidivist alcoholism. *Lancet* 1(8652):1435–1439.

This article presents one of the few controlled studies of the efficacy of acupuncture in the treatment of alcoholism. The study used forty treatment patients and forty controls all of whom received regular acupuncture "treatment." However, the patients received acupuncture at points that were specific for substance abuse while the control group patients received acupuncture at nonspecific points. The study group was much more likely to complete the acupuncture treatment than those in the control group, only one of whom completed the treatment. The results showed acupuncture to be effective in treating severe alcoholics, and the authors suggest that a further benefit of such treatment is that it avoids such patients being treated at expensive treatment centers.

Clement-Jones, V., Lowry, P. J., McLoughlin, L., et al. (1979). Acupuncture in heroin addicts: changes in met-enkephalin and beta-endorphin in blood and cerebrospinal fluid. *Lancet* 2(8139):380–382.

Equinox Group (1988). The equinox system and heroin addiction—mechanisms implicated in the application of acupuncture, electroacupuncture and electrostimulation for drug withdrawal. *Equinox Review* 4:1–4.

Jaffee, J. H. (1977). Some reflections on the evolution of current American approaches to problems of drug abuse and to the treatment of drug abusers. *Journal of Drug Issues* 7(1):1–12.

Lau, M. P. (1976). Acupuncture and addiction: an overview. *Addictive Diseases: An International Journal* 2(3):449–463.

Margolin, A., Change, P., Avants, S. K., and Kosten, T. R. (1993). Effects of sham and real auricular needling: implications for trials of acupuncture for cocaine addiction. *American Journal of Chinese Medicine* 21(2):103–111.

McDonald, D. (1990). Ayurveda and acupuncture in heroin detoxification in Sri Lanka. *Drug and Alcohol Review* 9:329–31.

McLellan, A. T., Grossman, D. S., Blaine, J. D., and Haverkos, H. W. (1993). Acupuncture treatment for drug abuse: a technical review. *Journal of Substance Abuse Treatment* 10:569–76.

Newmeyer, J. A., Johnson, G., and Klot, S. (1984). Acupuncture as a detoxification modality. *Journal of Psychoactive Drugs* 16(3):241–261.

The article concerns an eighteen-month study (from October 1979 to April 1981) on the efficacy of acupuncture in the detoxification on 297 heroin abusers treated at the Haight-Ashbury Free Medical Clinic, which was "one of the first American health agencies to employ acupuncture in the treatment of drug addiction" (p. 241). Patients "received 30 minute sessions of electrostimulation acupuncture, administered primarily in the 'lung' and 'God's door' ear points.... After an average of 12 acupuncture treatments, patients were free of most of the characteristic symptoms of addiction" (p. 241). Patients indicated that both the level of anxiety as well as their cravings for drugs had been significantly reduced. Those who completed the acupuncture treatment, however, were older and "were markedly more likely to have attended college, to be employed and to be only occasional heroin users" (p. 253) than the majority of patients. In one sense it served best those patients who least needed it. It was also found that most patients considered acupuncture to be foreign and to clash with what was considered appropriate treatment. Another inhibitor was that the effect of acupuncture was cumulative and despite providing improvements in symptoms and mood states it did not provide a quick relief or instant gratification. Thus, while the promise of acupuncture was considerable in the early 1980s at the Haight-Ashbury clinic it was found to fall considerably short of that promise.

Newmeyer, J. A., and Whitehead, C. (1977). Acupuncture and heroin addiction: a summary of the experience of the Haight-Ashbury Free Medical Clinic. In *A Multicultural View of Drug Abuse—Proceedings of the National Drug Abuse Conference, 1977*, ed. D. E. Smith, S. M. Anderson, M. Buxton, et al., pp. 404–409. Boston: Schenkman.

Patterson, M. A. (1975). *Addictions Can Be Cured—The Treatment of Drug Addiction by Neuro-Electric Stimulation.* Berhamsted, Hertfordshire, UK: Lion.

―― (1993). Neuroelectric therapy (NET) in addictions. *Neuroelectric Therapy*, pp. 1-4. Manuscript. Glasgow: NET.

Patterson, M. A., Patterson, L., Flood, N. V., et al. (1993). Electrostimulation in drug and alcohol detoxification—significance of stimulation criteria in clinical success. *Addiction Research* 1:130-144.

This article argues that it is the electrostimulation and its specific parameter, rather than the acupuncture per se, that is the deciding factor in the successful detoxification of addicts. Reference is made to three studies (in England, France, and Russia) that independently came to this conclusion, namely that "the clearly expressed therapeutic effect appears only if that frequency of pulse current is applied, which produces maximal brain beta-endorphin secretion" (p. 135). The specific frequency necessary is determined by the substance of addiction as well as the specific biochemistry of the addict.

Patterson and colleagues, while recognizing that acupuncture "can be effectively used as a support system for recovering drug abusers" (p. 138), claim that acupuncture per se, without electric stimulation, does not lead to rapid detoxification. Dr. Patterson was a colleague of Dr. Wen in Hong Kong in the early 1970s when he discovered the potential use of acupuncture for treating opium addicts.

Riet, G. T., Kleijnen, J., and Knipschild, P. (1990). A meta-analysis of studies into the effect of acupuncture on addiction. *British Journal of General Practice* 40(338):379-382.

This article presents a recent review of controlled clinical studies on the efficacy of acupuncture in the treatment of smoking, heroin, and alcohol addiction. Only a total of twenty-two such studies could be found and evaluated.

The authors found that more than half of the studies on smoking cessation had negative rather than positive outcomes. The authors assert that there are very few controlled clinical studies concerning heroin and alcohol addiction and that most of those that have been carried out are of low quality. "Claims that acupuncture is efficacious as a therapy for these addictions are thus not supported by results from sound clinical research" (p. 379). However, they do refer positively to the study by Bullock and colleagues (1989), which showed acupuncture to be efficacious in the treatment of alcohol addiction.

Schuckit, M. A. (1993). Acupuncture and the treatment of drug withdrawal syndromes. *Drug Abuse and Alcoholism Newsletter* 21:1–4.

Smith, M. O. (1988a). Acupuncture treatment for crack: clinical survey of 1,500 patients treated. *American Journal of Acupuncture* 16(3):241–247.

This is a study of crack addicts who received acupuncture treatment at the Lincoln Hospital drug addiction treatment program in New York City. "Each crack client averages four and one-half visits during the first month after intake. Less than 20 percent drop out after the initial visit. During Jan. 1987, 20 percent of the clients who began the program went on to give an average of ten clean urines each" (p. 242). Although this is not a particularly impressive result, Dr. Smith suggests that "the results become much more significant when it is noted that they describe success rates obtained on an unscreened population in an understaffed outpatient setting" (p. 243). He does not claim that acupuncture alone can successfully treat crack abusers but that with counseling it does seem to be a significant treatment component.

―――― (1988b). The Lincoln Hospital Acupuncture Drug Abuse Program—Testimony presented to Andrew Stein, President of the New York City Council (June 29).

Smith, M. O., and Khan, I. (1988). An acupuncture programme for the treatment of drug-addicted persons. *Bulletin on Narcotics* 40(1):35–41.

Washburn, A. M., Fullilove, R. E., Fullilove, M. T., et al. (1993). Acupuncture heroin detoxification: a single-blind clinical trial. *Journal of Substance Abuse Treatment* 10:345–351.

Wen, H. L. (1980). Clinical experience and mechanism of acupuncture and electrical stimulation (AES) in the treatment of drug abuse. *American Journal of Chinese Medicine* 8(4):349–353.

Wen, H. L., and Cheung, S. Y. C. (1973). Treatment of drug addiction by acupuncture and electrical stimulation. *Asian Journal of Medicine* 9:138–141.

This is the article that first brought attention to the possibility of the efficacy of acupuncture in the treatment of addicts. The work of Wen and Cheung is what eventually influenced the use of acupuncture for such treatment throughout the world. As they describe it:

> A new approach to relieving the drug withdrawal syndrome and counteracting drug addiction itself has been made at the Tung Wah and Kwong Wah hospitals, Hong Kong. The use of acupuncture and electrical stimulation for the dual purpose has been successfully tried for the first time. In this article, the authors report treating 40 cases of addiction (30 opium and 10 heroin) by the new method, and the relief of withdrawal symptoms and the degree of "drug-freedom" obtained. [p. 138]

The authors claim that the patients not only reported that they were free of symptoms but also that they felt good and were alert and relaxed.

The acupuncture sessions usually lasted 30 minutes each, although some patients required up to 45 minutes. Although they present their result in a very positive light they are also cautious in terms of cure, which they do not mention. They indicate that it is not until sixty days after treatment that a patient can begin to be declared drug free, and this still does not assure full rehabilitation.

Whitehead, P. C. (1978). Acupuncture in the treatment of addiction: a review and analysis. *International Journal of the Addictions* 13(1):1-16.

This is one of the first critical reviews of the efficacy of acupuncture in the treatment of addicts. "The use of acupuncture in the management of addictions are reviewed and found to fall seriously short of adequate clinical trials. The utility of acupuncture remains unproven" (p. 1). This was one of the precursors to the study carried out by Riet and colleagues (1990).

Worner, T. M., Zeller, B., Schwarz, H., et al. (1992). Acupuncture fails to improve treatment outcome in alcoholics. *Drug and Alcohol Dependence* 30:169-173.

Yang, M. M. P., and Kwok, J. S. L. (1986). Evaluation on the treatment of morphine addiction by acupuncture, Chinese herbs and opioid peptides. *American Journal of Chinese Medicine* 14(1-2):46-50.

2
Affect/Psychology/Behavior

Corcoran, J. P., and Longo, E. D. (1992). Psychological treatment of anabolic-androgenic steroid-dependent individuals. *Journal of Substance Abuse Treatment* 9:229–235.

Frye, R. V. (1990). Affective modes in multimodality addiction treatment. In *Treatment Choices for Alcoholism and Substance Abuse*, ed. H. B. Milkman and L. I. Sederer, pp. 287–307. Lexington, MA: Lexington Books.

The article implies that we all have a need, at times, to achieve a state of altered consciousness, but the author suggests that there are other ways than the use of drugs to do so such as "hiking in the wilderness . . . visiting a city . . . having sex, daydreaming, watching fireworks . . . participating in religious rituals" (p. 287). It would be desirable if, through such means, recovering addicts could self-regulate endogenous systems to produce what the author calls "natural highs." "Successful treatment leading to cessation of that addictive behavior must consist of training in other, less destructive ways of coping" (p. 288). The author suggests that there are many means by which this could be achieved, including "stress management training, meditation, biofeedback, creative therapies, charismatic group therapy, suggestion, and group marathon therapy, among others" (p. 291). The article discusses these different methods. Without expressing it in this way the author seems to suggest that, in addition to "saying no to drugs," people can also "say yes to natural highs," and to learn how these can be achieved in nondamaging ways.

Higgins, S. T., Delancy, D. D., Budney, A. J., et al. (1991). A behavioral approach to achieving initial cocaine abstinence. *American Journal of Psychiatry* 148(9):1218–1224.

3
ASC/Hallucinogens/High Mind

Allen, J. W., and Merlin, M. D. (1992). Psychoactive mushroom use in Koh Samui and Koh Pha-Ngan, Thailand. *Journal of Ethnopharmacology* 35:205–228.

Blum, K., and Tilton, J. E. (1981). Understanding the high mind. In *Folk Medicine and Herbal Healing*, ed. G. G. Meyer, K. Blum, and J. G. Cull, pp. 261–274. Springfield, IL: Charles C Thomas.

The authors suggest that the "Western world is left-hemisphere oriented" (p. 264). And the use of mind altering drugs may simply be a "unconscious" need to "simply suppress the left hemisphere and permit the stars to come out" (p. 265). The authors suggest that all people, including Westerners, do at times need, or at least desire to, reach a "high" state.

They go on to suggest that it is not basically "getting high" or even drug abuse that is the major problem, but rather loneliness and alienation, which can be seen as precursors to addiction. And thus they suggest that we all need (different) ways of achieving happiness and euphoria, and that various activities can stimulate endogenous biochemicals that allow us to reach such states without the use of exogenously ingested or injected drugs. "It is being demonstrated in laboratories today that there are naturally occurring substances floating around in the brain which have been identified as polypeptide material (endorphins) which are opiate-like in biological action and may induce euphoric states. These substances have been found to bind to the 'opiate receptor' in the brain as well as in the peripheral nervous system and produce analgesia (pain relief) and physical dependence much as do alcohol and morphine" (p. 271).

Bourguignon, E. (1977). Altered states of consciousness, myths, and rituals. In *Drugs, Rituals and Altered States of Consciousness*, ed. B. M. DuToit, pp. 7–23. Rotterdam: A. A. Balkema.

The author states that in most traditional societies altered states of consciousness (ASC) are usually part of the spiritual system. Of 488 societies studied, "ASCs were institutionalized within a religious framework in 90% of these" (p. 9). A number of means are used to achieve ASCs, including "drumming and singing and active dancing . . . [and] other means such as rhythmic sounds and motions, physical exertion, including dancing of whirling type, leading to a degree of disorientation, possibly also involving hyperventilation, suggestion, and concentration" (p. 10). The article discusses some of the differences between African and AmerIndian ASCs, with possession trance being more common in Africa than that of trance predominating in the Americas. Thus, there is also a much greater reliance on drugs in the Americas than in Africa. This makes sense since "possession trance requires greater awareness of the physical environment and of body coordination, to be able to act out the role of the spirits, as in dancing. . . . It may well be that drug use is relatively rare in Sub-Saharan African religious ritual, at least compared with the Americas" (p. 15).

ASCs occur in all human societies. They are very frequently embedded into religious patterns of belief and ceremonial, with varying degrees of ritualization. They are also very often ritualized in a secular context. Ritualization may be thought of as an imposition of order, a bringing under social and ideological control of what are potentially disruptive psychological states and forces. The very frequency of ritualization of ASCs suggests that in most societies many kinds of such states are so viewed, in a traditional sacred context, as well as in a modern secular one. [p. 21]

Brown, K. L. (1984). Hallucinogenic mushrooms, jade, obsidian, and the Guatemalan Highlands: What did the Olmecs really want? In *Trade and Exchange in Early Mesoamerica*, ed. K. G. Hirth, pp. 215–233. Albuquerque: University of New Mexico Press.

DeRios, M. D. (1986). Enigma of drug-induced altered states of consciousness among the !Kung Bushmen of the Kalahari Desert. *Journal of Ethnopharmacology* 15:297–304.

DuToit, B. M., ed. (1977). Introduction. In *Drugs, Rituals and Altered States of Consciousness*, pp. 1–4. Rotterdam: A. A. Balkema.

Kurland, A. A., Unger, S., Shaffer, J. W., and Savage, C. (1967). Psychedelic therapy utilizing LSD in the treatment of the alcoholic patient: a preliminary report. *American Journal of Psychiatry* 123(10):1202–1209.

LaBarre, W. (1975). Anthropological perspectives on hallucination and hallucinogens. In *Hallucinations: Behavior, Experience and Theory*, ed. R. K. Siegel, and L. J. West, pp. 9–52. New York: Wiley.

The author suggests that "every established religion began as a 'crisis cult,' when contemporary secular culture failed to provide resolution of overwhelming anxieties" (p. 22).

But in addition to religion (and as a part of religious experience) "there appears to be no human society so simple in material culture as to lack some sort of mood-altering drug as an escape from the workaday world" (p. 24). The article goes on to provide the examples of how different hallucinogenic substances have been (and are) used in different parts of the world.

Lee, R. L. M. (1989). Self-presentation in Malaysian spirit seances: a dramaturgical perspective on altered states of consciousness in healing ceremonies. In *Altered States of Consciousness and Mental Health—A Cross-Cultural Perspective*, Cross-Cultural Research and Methodology Series, vol. 12, ed. C. A. Ward, pp. 251–266. Newbury Park, CA: Sage.

Lemlij, M. (1978). Primitive group treatment. *Psychiatria Clinics* 11:10–14.

McPeake, J. D., Kennedy, B. P., and Gordon, S. M. (1991). Altered states of consciousness therapy—A missing component in alcohol and drug rehabilitation treatment. *Journal of Substance Abuse Treatment* 8:75–82.

This article posits that achieving altered states of consciousness is a basic human motive. The authors suggest that there is a growing body of literature that supports the benefits derived from achieving ASC and that drug rehabilitation treatment programs' failure to consider this may be linked to their high failure rates. "Most such programs make little or no effort to systematically expose patients to constructive alternative methods for experiencing nonordinary consciousness" (p. 76). However, by pointing out that an organization such as Alcoholics Anonymous encourages its members to seek a change in consciousness and to achieve a "spiritual awakening," the authors support their argument that the consideration of ASCs is not esoteric or "strange" and should be central to addict rehabilitation programs.

The article describes an altered states of consciousness therapy (ASCT) program that can be used "to teach patients to consciously manipulate affect and cognition to achieve a new consciousness."

Pigot, R. (1975). The concept of altered states of consciousness and how it helps us understand the drug scene. *Medical Journal of Australia* 2(23):882–884.

This article states that despite material wealth people are increasingly realizing the poverty of their lives and many seek a solution through the use of drugs. The author suggests that a way of combatting drug abuse is through helping each other discover the natural "highs" derived from the fundamental aspects of being human.

Roy, S., and Rizvi, S. H. M. (1987). Tribal hallucinogenic tradition: a case study of Manipur village. *Man in India* 87(2):137–146.

Schultes, R. E. (1984). Fifteen years of study of psychoactive snuffs of South America: 1967–1982—a review. *Journal of Ethnopharmacology* 11:17–32.

Valla, J.-P., and Prince, R. H. (1989). Religious experiences as self-healing mechanisms. In *Altered States of Consciousness and Mental Health—A Cross-Cultural Perspective*, Cross-Cultural Research and Methodology Series, vol. 12, ed. C. A. Ward, pp. 149–166. Newbury Park, CA: Sage.

Based on a study of upper-middle class Americans, this chapter proposes that religious experiences trigger endogenous healing mechanisms, bringing about self-healing and resistance to alcohol abuse.

Ward, C. A. (1989). The cross-cultural study of altered states of consciousness and mental health. In *Altered States of Consciousness and Mental Health—A Cross-Cultural Perspective*, Cross-Cultural Research and Methodology Series, vol. 12, ed. C. A. Ward, pp. 15–35. Newbury Park, CA: Sage.

———, ed. (1989). *Altered States of Consciousness and Mental Health—A Cross-Cultural Perspective*, Cross-Cultural Research and Methodology Series, vol. 12. Newbury Park, CA: Sage.

4
Biofeedback/Relaxation

Brinkman, D. N. (1978). Biofeedback application to drug addiction in the University of Colorado drug rehabilitation program. *International Journal of the Addictions* 13(5):817–830.

Brown, B. (1975). Biofeedback: an exercise in "self-control." *Saturday Review*, February 22, pp. 22–26.

This article concludes:

> Biofeedback has been successful in an unbelievable array of problems of health: tension and migraine headaches, cardiac irregularities, high blood pressure, peripheral vascular disease, gastric ulcer, insomnia, epilepsy, asthma, spastics, learning problems in children, and a host of other troublesome medical and psychological problems in human beings. And along the way it is opening the door to a more holistic approach to therapy. [p. 26]

Denney, M. R., Baugh, J. L., and Hardt, H. D. (1991). Sobriety outcome after alcoholism treatment with biofeedback participation: a pilot inpatient study. *International Journal of the Addictions* 26(3):335–341.

This article confirms previous results about the relevance of biofeedback in alcoholism treatment. Biofeedback was found significant in maintaining sobriety, but the authors suggest that optimal results are achieved if patients have at least six biofeedback training sessions.

Klajner, F., Hartman, L. M., and Sobell, M. B. (1984). Treatment of substance abuse by relaxation training: a review of its rationale, efficacy and mechanisms. *Addictive Behaviors* 9:41–55.

Lamontagne, Y., Hand, I., Annable, L., and Gagnon, M.-A. (1975). Physiological and psychological effects of alpha and EMG feedback training with college drug users. A pilot study. *Canadian Psychiatric Association Journal* 20(5):337–348.

Roszell, D. K., and Chaney, E. F. (1982). Autogenic training in a drug abuse program. *International Journal of Addictions* 17(8):1337–1349.

5
Various Countries/Thailand/ Southeast Asia

Arokiasamy, C. M. V., and Taricone, P. T. (1992). Drug rehabilitation in West Malaysia: an overview of its history and development. *International Journal of the Addictions* 27(11):1301–1311.

Baasher, T. A., and Abu El Azayem, G. M. (1980). Egypt: the role of the mosque in treatment. In *Drug Problems in Sociocultural Context—A Basis for Policies and Programme Planning*, Public Health Paper no.73, ed. G. Edwards and A. Arif, pp. 131–134. Geneva:WHO.

This article describes the involvements of sheikhs at a number of mosques in Egypt engaged in the treatment of addicts. Of the 4,000 mosques in Cairo alone, some 400 were involved in addict rehabilitation at the time of this article, and it is expected that many more can be convinced to join in this work. Treatment at these mosques is quite popular, with many more addicts seeking treatment there than at the more orthodox (and official) rehabilitation programs. Treatment at the mosques costs about nine American dollars, which was less than half of the cost of treatment elsewhere in Cairo.

Chandrasena, R. (n.d.). Opium dependence following treatment—"traditional practitioners" in Sri Lanka. Unpublished manuscript.

deSilva, P. (1983). The Buddhist attitude to alcoholism. In *Drug Use and Misuse—Cultural Perspectives* (Based on a Collaborative Study by the World Health Organization), ed. G. Edwards, A. Arif, and J. Jaffe, pp. 33–41. London: Croom Helm.

> Interestingly, and perhaps predictably, the individual victim of alcoholism is treated with sympathy and tolerance by the religious order.... This is partly due to the overall attitude of tolerance in Buddhism, which considers 'metta,' or living kindness, as an ideal. [p. 40]

Edwards, G. (1983). Countries differ in their treatment of drug problems. In *Drug Use and Misuse—Cultural Perspectives* (Based on a Collaborative Study by the World Health Organization), ed. G. Edwards, A. Arif, and J. Jaffe, pp. 176–184. London: Croom Helm.

Edwards, G., and Arif, A. (1983). The future. In *Drug Use and Misuse—Cultural Perspectives* (Based on a Collaborative Study by the World Health Organization), ed. G. Edwards, A. Arif, and J. Jaffe, pp. 269–274. London: Croom Helm.

> The argument throughout this book has been that it is impossible to think about, or constructively respond to, any aspect of drug-taking without, at every stage, seeing drug-taking in its socio-cultural context. [p. 269]

> What is needed rather is the further development of a model that would see treatment as a partnership between the individual, the community and the helping professions, with the helping professions in an assistant role. [p. 272]

It must be hoped that in the future there will be much more open exchange of ideas than has sometimes been seen, with no one dominant cultural view. This is a vital consideration equally for treatment, preventive action and research. Drugs are again only the exemplar of wider problems, and at worst of the general belief that if foreigners are not like us, they are wrong. [p. 274]

The authors conclude by urging that we listen to and learn from the experiences in a variety of countries; the way forward to more effective treatment programs lies in the sharing of such experiences.

Edwards, G., Arif, A., and Jaffe, J. (1983). *Drug Use and Misuse— Cultural Perspectives* (Based on a Collaborative Study by the World Health Organization). London: Croom Helm.

Giannini, A. J., Miller, N. S., and Turner, C. E. (1992). Treatment of Khat addiction. *Journal of Substance Abuse Treatment* 9:379–382.

Jilek-Aall, L., and Jilek, W. G. (1985). Buddhist temple treatment of narcotic addiction and neurotic-psychosomatic disorders in Thailand. In *Psychiatry: The State of the Art*, vol. 8, ed. P. P. Berner, R. Wolf, et al., pp. 673–677. New York: Plenum.

This article describes the addict treatment program at Wat Tam Krabok (Tham Krabok temple, about 100 miles north of Bangkok) and at a number of other Buddhist temples in Thailand. The Wat Tam Krabok rehabilitation program was established by nine Tudong monks in 1957 and by 1963 it had already earned a wide reputation for treating opium addicts. The abbot, Mr. Pra Cham-Roon, a former Bangkok police officer, used his knowledge of the plight of addicts obtained from his previous work, and was a significant figure in the development of this program, which "combined application of Buddhist philosophy and indigenous herbal and physical therapy" (p. 74).

By the time of this article, "50,000 Thai drug addicts as well as a few from Western countries" had been treated. "The treatment is dramatic and involves physical stress.... [The ingestion of a '100 herbs' concoction is] supposed to clear the drug residues from the body by inducing violent vomiting and diarrhea.... The patients' retching and moaning is accompanied by loud rhythmic drumming." The patients are then urged to drink a great deal of water and to take "regular steam baths with herbal ingredients" (p. 74) and to do physical exercise. The program uses death and rebirth symbolism, with the patient being stripped of his old clothes and personal belongings and putting on a new garment. But unlike a number of other death and rebirth programs the patient is treated as a prospective equal and it maintains the addict's human dignity.

Johnson, S. H. (1983). Treatment of drug abusers in Malaysia: a comparison. *International Journal of the Addictions* 18 (7):951–958.

Lee, R. L. M. (1985). Alternative systems in Malaysian drug rehabilitation: organization and control in comparative perspective. *Social Science and Medicine* 21(11):1289–1296.

Mala, T. A. (1985). Alcoholism and mental health treatment in circumpolar areas: traditional and non-traditional approaches. *Circumpolar Health* 84:332–334.

This article describes the spirit movement of the Northwest Alaska Native Association (NANA) and its approach in treating alcoholics.

"The Spirit Movement is basically a philosophy which stresses self responsibility and concern for those around us.... Using basic Inupiaq (Eskimo) values and having its roots in the community itself, it is a movement from within this Native society to improve itself and bring itself closer together in response to the increasing rate of alcoholism, suicide, and mental health problems" (p. 333). It is based on a belief that true change must come from within.

> The Spirit Movement has a set of basic values for Native People that include sharing, caring for others, responsibility for self, knowledge of language and traditions, pride in one's heritage, respect for elders and an inclusion of them in daily lives.
> A "spirit camp" has been established where there are no telephones or modern conveniences and where young people can go back to traditional hunting and fishing methods as passed on there by the elders.
> Native healers are employed to work with modern-day medical personnel. Traditional modern-day methods of healing such as body manipulation, massage, use of hot springs, Native herbs, and community support are stressed.
> The Spirit Movement program does not support an unrealistic "going back" to an earlier time of life.... It does advocate looking towards the elements of strength and spirituality that have sustained these peoples throughout the centuries as a way of surviving this cultural shock and combatting the trend toward cultural assimilation. [p. 334]

McGovern, M. P. (1982). Alcoholism in Southeast Asia—prevalence and treatment. *International Journal of Psychiatry* 28:36–44.

Poshyachinda, V. (1980). Thailand: treatment at the Tam Kraborg Temple. In *Drug Problems in Sociocultural Context—A Basis* for Policies and Programme Planning, Public Health Paper no. 73, ed. G. Edwards and A. Arif, pp. 121–125. Geneva: WHO.

—— (1982). *Indigenous drug dependence treatment in Thailand.* Paper presented at the 7th meeting of ASEAN (Association of Southeast Asian Nations) drug experts, Pattaya, Thailand, November–December.

—— (1984). Indigenous treatment for drug dependence in Thailand. *Impact of Science on Society* (no. 133) 34(1):67–76.

—— (1993). *A review on the Buddhist temple drug dependence treatment in Thailand.* Paper presented at the meeting of WHO Substance Abuse Collaborating Centres, Geneva, September.

This article reviews the therapeutic work done at the Wat Tam Kraborg and a number of other Buddhist temples, such as those at Wat Sri Soda, Wat Pay Pang in Chiang Mai Province, Tam Talu Centre, and Wat Tha Shee Srisumungklaram. The treatment of opium addiction has a long history in Thailand and in 1908 there were records of traditional herbal treatments that were claimed to be effective in treating as well as preventing opium smoking.

The treatment regimen instituted by the Tam Kraborg Temple treatment program is said to have been originally started by a nun in Saraburi Province who had inherited knowledge of herbal medicine. She conducted a trial of herbal medicine for opium dependence treatment leading to the therapy that was consequently used by her nephew, abbot Pra Chamroon Parnchan.

San Pedro, R. M., and Ponce, E. G. (1988). School programmes in drug rehabilitation and social reintegration in the Philippines. *Bulletin on Narcotics* 40(1):63–66.

Schuckit, M. A. (1989). Kava. *Drug Abuse and Alcoholism Newsletter* 18(2):1–3.

Sharma, K., and Shukla, V. (1988). Rehabilitation of drug-addicted persons: the experience of the Nav-Chetna Center in India. *Bulletin on Narcotics* 40(1):43–49.

The Nav-Chetna Drug De-addiction and Rehabilitation Center in Varanasi was established in December 1985. It provided therapy by means of counseling, educational and vocational guidance, yoga therapy and after care. Yoga played a particularly important role in both the pre- and post-clinical stages, "to promote personal development, to build up and strengthen their initiative and confidence and to bring about improvement in their maturation, attitude and behaviors to overcome addiction . . . self-actualize."

The authors state that "motivation to abandon drug addiction is perhaps the single most important factor for successful rehabilitation" (p. 44). As have a number of other articles, this one claims that "in order for drug abuse programmes to be effective, they must provide a non-chemical alternative that can offset at least some of the motivations to abuse drugs."

"The approach . . . is to build up individual motivation and initiative . . . creating physical and psychological conditions that optimize the natural tendency of the individual's system to self-actualize and eventually stabilize" (p. 44). "Yoga, as a system for rejuvenation, becomes a natural ally, offering a systematic method of achieving this goal in a relatively short period of time" (p. 45). During the period 1986–88, about 1,700 persons underwent treatment for drug addiction. "Life became more fulfilling with the daily practice of yoga. . . . When detoxification began, individuals were already highly motivated" (p. 48).

Shrestha, N. M. (1992). Alcohol and drug abuse in Nepal. *British Journal of Addiction* 87:1241–1248.

Suwaki, H. (1980). Japan: culturally based treatment of alcoholism. In *Drug Problems in Sociocultural Context—A Basis for Policies and Programme Planning*, Public Health Paper no. 73, ed. G. Edwards and A. Arif, pp. 139–143. Geneva: WHO.

> Alcoholics Anonymous, which is popular in the West, is found in only limited areas of Japan. But . . . Danshukai (Alcohol Abstinence Society) is widespread throughout Japan. As for individual therapy, psychoanalysis and behavioral therapy are rarely used with Japanese alcoholics, but supportive and educational therapies are being offered by interested therapists. Naikan therapy (self-observation psychotherapy) is one of these. It has its origin in Japanese Buddhism, and it is effectively practiced with Japanese alcoholics." [p. 140]

Danshukai: "Twenty-five thousand members were attending the meetings in 1977, and 16,000 had abstained from alcohol over one year" (p. 140).

Suwanwela, C., and Poshyachinda, V. (1983). Thailand: rendering opium redundant. In *Drug Use and Misuse—Cultural Perspectives* (Based on a Collaborative Study by the World Health Organization), ed. G. Edwards, A. Arif, and J. Jaffe, pp. 215–220. London: Croom Helm.

—— (1986). Drug abuse in Asia. *Bulletin on Narcotics* 38 (1, 2):41–53.

U Khant (1985). Measures to prevent and reduce drug abuse among young people in Burma. *Bulletin on Narcotics* 37 (2, 3):81–89.

Westermeyer, J. (1973). Folk treatment for opium addiction in Laos. *British Journal of Addiction* 68:345–349.

——— (1979). Medical and nonmedical treatment for narcotic addicts—a comparative study from Asia. *Journal of Nervous and Mental Disease* 167(4):205–211.

6

Herbal Treatment

Nebelkopf, E. (1987). Herbal therapy in the treatment of drug use. *International Journal of Addictions* 22(8):695–717.

—— (1988). Herbs and substance abuse treatment: a 10-year perspective. *Psychoactive Drugs* 20(3):349–354.

This article begins by stating, "There is a growing awareness of and concern to develop programs for substance abusers which utilize a holistic approach to deal with the mental, physical, emotional and spiritual problems accompanying substance abuse" (p. 695). It then goes on to suggest that people take drugs in order to feel better, and that one of the solutions to the problem of drug abuse involves creating opportunities for people to experience nonchemical alternatives. The author suggests, "Herbs provide a meaningful alternative for drug abusers and the use of herbs reflects a paradigm shift in life-style and self-concept away from the self-application of chemicals" (p. 696).

Shanmugasundaram, E. R. B., and Shanmugasundaram, K. R. (1986). An Indian herbal formula (SKY) for controlling voluntary ethanol intake in rats with chronic alcoholism. *Journal of Ethnopharmacology* 17:171–182.

Yang, M. M. P., Yuen, R. C. F., and Kwok, J. S. L. (1985). Effect of certain Chinese herbs on drug addiction. In *Advances in Chinese Medicinal Materials Research*, ed. H. M. Chang, H. W. Yeung, W. W. Tso, and A. Koo, pp. 147–158. Singapore: World Scientific Press.

The authors report on the use of Chinese herbs in a study of 300 cases of opium and heroin addicts in Hong Kong in which it was found that the herbs Qiang Huo, Gou Teng, Chuan Ziong, Fu Zi, and Yan Hu Suo significantly reduced withdrawal symptoms.

7

Ibogaine

Cappendijk, S. L. T., and Dzoljic, M. R. (1993). Inhibitory effects of ibogaine on cocaine self-administration in rats. *European Journal of Pharmacology* 241:261–265.

Cowley, G., Heiman, H., and Ramo, J. C. (1993). A psychedelic trip to the end of addiction. *Newsweek* 122(8):45.

Deecher, D. C., Teitler, M., Soderlund, D. M., et al. (1992). Mechanisms of action of ibogaine and harmaline congeners based on radioligand binding studies. *Brain Research* 571:242–247.

This article suggest that the ibogaine might be effective in the treatment of drug addicts, but that further studies are needed.

> Long-lasting, dose-dependent behavioral effects of ibogaine have been reported. The possibility that these effects were due to irreversible binding properties of ibogaine at K-receptors was considered; however, radioligand wash experiments showed a rapid recovery of radioligand binding after one wash. . . . In summary, the results of our study indicate that ibogaine analogs show affinity for the K-opiate receptor. The action of ibogaine, or an active metabolite, at this receptor may be responsible for its putative anti-addictive properties. [p. 246]

Fernandez, J. W. (1972). Tabernanthe Iboga: narcotic ecstases and the work of ancestors. In *Flesh of the Gods—The Ritual Use of Hallucinogens*, ed. P. Furst, pp. 237–260. New York: Praeger.

> This is an extensive chapter concerning the traditional ritual use of ibogaine (or Tabernanthe iboga—*eboka* in the local language) in the all-night ceremonies by the Bwiti cult of Gabon, West Africa. Through the use of *eboka* ritual participants are able "to maintain a high level of engagement in the ritual development over a long period of time without complaint or fatigue." However, the author also suggests, "the beauty and integration achieved in this cult by dance and song are virtually sufficient in themselves to achieve euphoric results, even without 'eboka'" (p. 255).

Glick, S. D., Gallagher, C. A., Hough, L. B., et al. (1992). Differential effects of ibogaine pretreatment on brain levels of morphine and (+)amphetamine. *Brain Research* 588:173–176.

Glick, S. D., Rossman, K., Steindorf, S., et al. (1991). Effects and aftereffects of ibogaine on morphine self-administration in rats. *European Journal of Pharmacology* 195:341–345.

> Ibogaine, a naturally occurring alkaloid, has been claimed to be effective in treating addiction to opiate and stimulant drugs. As a preclinical test of this claim, the present study sought to determine if ibogaine would reduce the intravenous self-administration of morphine in rats. Ibogaine dose dependently (2.5–80 mg/kg) decreased morphine intake in the hour after ibogaine treatment. . . . In some rats, there was a persistent decrease in morphine intake for several days or weeks after a single injection of ibogaine. . . . Further studies are needed to characterize the nature of the ibogaine-morphine interaction as well as to determine if

ibogaine also affects the self-administration of other drugs. [p. 341]

Jeter, A. (1994). The psychedelic cure. *The New York Times Magazine*, April 10, pp. 50–52.

The author suggests that studies have shown that the use of ibogaine (Tabernanthe iboga) inhibits drug craving for many months, and sometimes for several years, and has the advantage over such therapies as methadone in that its use does not lead to another dependency.

However, the author also refers to Charles Grudzinskas, director of the medications development division of the NIDA, who, albeit interested in conducting further studies, states, "There is really no evidence that it works." Ibogaine "was an over-the-counter fatigue remedy in France into the 1960s. In the late 1960s researchers at the University of California at Berkeley reported another side of ibogaine: it unlocks repressed childhood memories" (p. 50). The article discusses its use by Lotsof in treating addicts in the Netherlands and also reports on the one fatality apparently associated with its use (no other fatality has been reported). The U. S. Food and Drug Administration in 1994 allowed two neuroscientists at the University of Miami, D. Mash and J. Sanchez-Ramos, to begin human tests on the efficacy of ibogaine in treating addicts.

Maisonneuve, I. M., and Glick, S. D. (1992). Interactions between ibogaine and cocaine in rats: in vivo microdialysis and motor behavior. *European Journal of Pharmacology* 212: 263–266.

Touchette, N. (1993). Ibogaine neurotoxicity raises new questions in addiction research. *Journal of NIH Research* 5:50–55.

The article begins by reporting on the use of the hallucinogenic plant ibogaine by a group of drug users in the 1960s, leading to the serious possibility that its use could be effective in the treatment of addiction to a range of substances. Recent research is discussed showing promising results. These have raised a number of questions about the efficacy and official use of ibogaine for addiction therapy, which led researchers to initiate new and more substantial scientific investigations.

8

Meditation/TM Treatment

Anderson, D. (1977). Transcendental meditation as an alternative to heroin abuse in service. *American Journal of Psychiatry* 134(11):1308–1309.

Benson, H., and Wallace, R. K. (1972). Decreased drug abuse with transcendental meditation—a study of 1,862 subjects. In *Drug Abuse: Proceedings of the International Conference*, ed. C. J. D. Zarafonetis, pp. 369–376. Philadelphia: Lea & Febiger.

Although the authors indicate that the efficacy of meditation programs in treating addicts had yet to be established, the study reported on here did indicate a significant reduction in drug taking associated with the practice of transcendental meditation.

> Questionnaires were given to approximately 1,950 subjects who had been practicing TM for three months or more and who were attending one of two meditation training courses offered by the Students' International Meditation Society in the summer of 1970. [p. 370]

> After starting TM there was a significant decrease in the amount of drugs used or discontinuance of drug use; a decrease or cessation in engaging in drug-selling activity; and

changed attitudes in the direction of discouraging others from abusing drugs. Further, the subjects decreased their consumption of "hard" alcoholic beverages and smoked fewer cigarettes. [p. 375]

Clements, G., Krenner, L., and Molk, W. (1988). The use of the transcendental meditation programme in the prevention of drug abuse and in the treatment of drug-addicted persons. *Bulletin on Narcotics* 40(1):51–56.

The authors suggest that the practice of transcendental meditation does not in itself constitute a rehabilitation programme but is rather a means of self-development. They suggest that many rehabilitation programmes fail when the external support of counselor, doctor, alternative drugs, and other factors are removed. They claim that therapeutic success is greatly dependent on the development of the individual's inner resources.

"To date, over 350 research studies have been conducted in research institutions in over 25 countries" (p. 52). The authors claim that there is now substantial evidence the 15 to 20 minutes of transcendental meditation practice twice a day is clearly associated with a significant reduction and abstinence of drug taking.

Galanter, M., and Buckley, P. (1978). Evangelical religion and meditation: psychotherapeutic effects. *Journal of Nervous and Mental Disease* 166(10):685–691.

Ganguli, H. C. (1985). Meditation subculture and drug use. *Human Relations* 38(10):953–962.

Gelderloos, P., Walton, K. G., Orrne-Johnson, D. W., and Alexander, C. N. (1991). Effectiveness of the transcendental meditation program in preventing and treating substance misuse: a review. *International Journal of Addictions* 26(3):293–325.

This article reports on a 1990 review of 24 studies, all of which showed a positive drug addiction therapeutic effect of the practice of transcendental meditation. While critically examining these studies and suggesting the need to view all the claims of efficacy with some skepticism, the authors do conclude that the practice of transcendental meditation does indeed have many positive results even if it cannot be claimed as a definitive treatment for addiction.

9

Other

Arredondo, R., Weddige, R. L., Justice, C. L., and Fitz, J. (1987). Alcoholism in Mexican-Americans: intervention and treatment. *Hospital and Community Psychiatry* 38(2):180–183.

Davis, W. (1985). Hallucinogenic plants and their use in traditional societies—an overview. *Cultural Survival Quarterly* 9(4):2–5.

> The passionate desire which leads man to flee from the monotony of everyday life has made him instinctively discover strange substances. He has done so, even where nature has been most niggardly in producing them and where the products seem very far from possessing the properties which would enable him to satisfy this desire. [p. 2]

Although drug users in Western urban societies also engage in some ritualistic drug taken activities the author suggests that the use of hallucinogenic plants in "traditional societies" was and is generally quite different from that occurring in more "cosmopolitan" societies, as may be noted by the following concluding sentences:

> The ceremonial use of hallucinogenic plants by the Amerindian is (most often) a collective journey into the unconscious. It is not necessarily, and in fact rarely is, a

pleasant or an easy journey. It is wondrous and it may be terrifying. But above all it is purposeful. . . . In eastern North America during puberty rites, the Algonquin confined adolescents to a longhouse for two weeks and fed them a beverage based in part on datura. During the extended intoxication and the subsequent amnesia—a pharmacological feature of this drug—the young boys forgot what it was to be a child so that they might learn what it meant to be a man. . . . The experience is explicitly sought for positive ends. It is not a means of escaping from an uncertain existence; rather it is perceived as a means of contributing to the welfare of all one's people. [p. 5]

Deitch, D., and Solit, R. (1993). International training for drug abuse treatment and the issue of cultural relevance. *Journal of Psychoactive Drugs* 25(1):87-95.

During the last ten years, there has been an increased demand for culturally relevant drug abuse treatment that is responsive to the unique needs of international populations, each with its own special culture and taboos. This article explores the assumptions that these distinct cultural characteristics require different treatment approaches to be effective, and presents both curriculum content and training designs used in educating diverse cultures in drug abuse treatment strategies. The authors discuss their training experiences in Central Europe, the Mediterranean, China, and Southeast Asian countries and conclude that, while cultural uniqueness certainly exist, it may be greatly exaggerated in terms of the need for special treatment modalities in the field of drug abuse treatment. [p. 87]

DeRios, M. D., and Smith, D. E. (1984). Drug use and abuse in cross-cultural perspective. In *Culture and Psychopathology*, ed. J. E. Mezzich, and C. E. Berganza, pp. 385-399. New York: Columbia University Press.

In reviewing data from 488 ["traditional"] societies it was shown that "90 percent reported to have one or more institutionalized, culturally patterned form of altered states of consciousness" (p. 386) and that such ritualized drug use did not threaten the societies at large nor harm the individuals involved.

"In those societies where plant hallucinogens have played a central role, ethnographers describe beliefs of the drug user that he can see, feel, touch, and experience the unknown.... The central commandment of such societies seems to be to make the secular sacred" (p. 394).

Hopson. J. L. (1988). A pleasurable chemistry. *Psychology Today*, July/August, pp. 29–33.

Ja, D. Y., and Aoki, B. (1993). Substance abuse treatment: cultural barriers in the Asian-American community. *Journal of Psychoactive Drugs* 25(1):61–71.

Johnson, R. E., Jaffe, R. H., and Fudala, P. J. (1992). A controlled trial of buprenorphine treatment for opioid dependence. *Journal of the American Medical Association* 267(20): 2750–2755.

Jonas, D. F., and Jonas, A. D. (1977). A bioanthropological overview of addiction. *Perspectives in Biology and Medicine* 20:345–354.

Lex, B. W. (1987). Review of alcohol problems in ethnic minority groups. *Journal of Consulting and Clinical Psychology* 55(3):293–300.

Lex, B. W., and Meyer, R. E. (1977). Opiate receptors and opiate antagonists: progress in the "war on drugs." *Journal of Drug Issues* 7(1):54–60.

"The 'War on Drugs' has spawned major research efforts that have led to the discovery of the 'opiate receptor' and the development of new narcotic antagonists which may be useful adjuncts in the rehabilitation of chronic opiate addicts. At the moment [1977], these findings are rich with potential applications and potential discovery. The authors review the current state of the art" (p. 54).

Although this article is now somewhat dated it was one of the first that discussed the significance of the opiate receptors and its stimulation in the treatment of addicts.

McLellan, A. T., Grissom, G. R., Brill, P., et al. (1993). Private substance abuse treatments: Are some programs more effective than others? *Journal of Substance Abuse Treatment* 10:243–254.

Miller, W. R. (1992). The effectiveness of treatment of substance abuse. *Journal of Substance Abuse Treatment* 9:93–102.

NADA (National Acupuncture Detoxification Association) (1990). Nada Pamphlet. New York: NADA.

Nathan, R. G., Robinson, D., Cherek, D. R., et al. (1986). Alternative treatments for withdrawing the long-term benzodiazepine user: a pilot study. *International Journal of the Addictions* 21(2):195–211.

Rowe, D., and Grills, C. (1993). An alternative conceptual paradigm for drug counseling with African-American clients. *Journal of Psychoactive Drugs* 25(1):21–33.

> An alternative conceptual framework is presented for understanding the culturally normative behavior of African-Americans in drug abuse treatment and recovery, based on an appreciation of core African-centered beliefs. Key ontological and epistemological assumptions of traditional clinical and counseling interventions are presented that highlight the differences between traditional goals and theories

and the proposed alternative conceptual system and treatment strategies. Implications for African-centered treatment and future research on the course of addiction and recovery among African-Americans are discussed. [p. 21]

The following passage was particularly noted:

> In current drug research there is no general theory to delineate the effects of racism on African-American patterns of drug abuse and recovery. Experiences of racial stress are commonly excluded from either measures of stress or variables examined as possible contributors to the variance observed in patterns of use and recovery. . . . Until the treatment system operates from a broader frame of reference . . . that validates the life experiences, culture, and daily realities of African-Americans, low utilization of services, high attrition rates and indifference to negative attributions of the drug treatment system will continue. [p. 30]

Smith, D. E., Buxton, M. E., Bilal, R., and Seymour, R. B. (1993). Cultural points of resistance to the 12-step recovery process. *Journal of Psychoactive Drugs* 25(1):97–108.

> This article addresses some of the key issues in developing culturally relevant approaches to drug abuse treatment and recovery, using the HAFC/Glide African-American Extended Family Program as a positive example of effective cultural adaptability within recovery. Cultural points of resistance to the recovery process are also addressed, including the perception that 12-step fellowships are exclusive and confused with religion, confusion over surrender versus powerlessness, and concerns about low self-esteem, dysfunctional family structure, communication difficulties, and institutionalized and internalized racism. The authors also focus on professional resistance in other countries, where different treatment approaches and philosophies block the acceptance of a recovery concept in general and the 12-step

process in particular. In explicating these issues, addiction is presented as a multicultural problem in need of multicultural solutions. The challenge is to adapt the process of recovery to all cultures and races, to counter stereotypes on all sides, and to eliminate the perception that recovery only works for addicts from the white mainstream. [p. 97]

Sorhaug, H. C. (1988). Identitet: Grenser, autonomi og avhengighet—Soffmisbruk som eksempel. [Identity: frontiers, autonomy and dependency—addiction as an example.] *Alkoholpolidk—Tidskrift for nordisk alkoholforskning* 5:31–39.

Westermeyer, J. (1989). Nontreatment factors affecting treatment outcome in substance abuse. *American Journal of Drug and Alcohol Abuse* 15(1):13–29.

Wilson, P. (1987). The understanding of drug use, abuse and dependence, and its treatment by homeopathy and other therapies. Unpublished manuscript.

Zweben, J. E., ed. (1993). Culturally relevant substance abuse treatment. *Journal of Psychoactive Drugs* 25(1):1–108.

10
Psychodrama/Art Therapy/ Music Therapy/Books

Barker, S. B., Horvatich, P. K., and Schnoll, S. H. (1995). The use of a single concept music intervention in substance abuse treatment: a preliminary study. *Substance Abuse* 14(1): 35–44.

Crawford, R. J. M. (1989). Follow up of alcohol and other drug dependents treated with psychodrama. *New Zealand Medical Journal* 102(866):199.

Dushman, R. D., and Bressler, M. J. (1991). Psychodrama in an adolescent chemical dependency treatment program. *Individual Psychology* 47(4):515–520.

Johnson, L. (1990). Creative therapies in the treatment of addictions: the art of transforming shame. *The Arts in Psychotherapy* 17:299–308.

> This is an excellent article discussing the use of creative drug addiction therapies, which also uses the concept of the "'wounded healer,' in the tradition of the shamanic, spiritual guide" (p. 299), which appears to be a particularly effective approach. Healing takes place through the creative process, that is, by listening to, commenting on, or writing a poem or engaging in other creative activities.

McDonald, E. (1985). Creative writing therapy used to assist chemically dependent adolescents express feelings. In *International Council on Alcohol and Addictions: Alcohol, Drugs and Tobacco*, pp. 130–132. Lausanne: ICAA.

Mahony, J., and Waller, D. (1992). Art therapy in the treatment of alcohol and drug abuse. In *Art Therapy: A Handbook*, ed. D. Waller, and A. Gilroy, pp. 173–188. Buckingham: Open University Press.

The article explores the possibility of art therapy's reducing resistance to therapy and enabling the addict to get in touch with his inner, or "authentic," self. By making art objects it is possible for the addict to express threatening materials about himself without experiencing the expected destruction of such a revelation.

The authors conclude:

> In this chapter, we have examined how art therapists approach working with clients who have problems with drugs and alcohol and how far they formulate their ideas with regard to theory and practice. It appears that art therapy has a unique contribution to make to this field in offering a vehicle for the exploration and expression of feelings that are experienced as overwhelming. However, it would seem from much of the literature that the majority do not relate their technique to their theoretical ideas; if this is a problem only with this particular client group, further research would need to be done to ascertain the reasons. [p. 187]

Pardeck, J. T. (1991). Using books to prevent and treat adolescent chemical dependency. *Adolescence* 26(101):201–208.

11
Ritual/Spiritism/Revivalism/ Spirituality in Treatment

Baer, H. A. (1981). Prophets and advisors in black spiritual churches: Therapy, palliative, or opiate? *Culture, Medicine and Psychiatry* 5:145–170.

This article examines a variant of Black ethnomedicine in urban areas, namely the complex of prophets and advisors found within the Spiritual movement. Based upon fieldwork among Spiritual churches in several cities and intensive interviews with Spiritual mediums in Nashville, Tennessee, attention is given to the form of folk psychotherapy that these prophets and advisors provide the members of their congregations as well as other individuals. Although it is argued that the complex of mediums in Black Spiritual churches provides an important coping mechanism for certain Blacks, it is important, particularly in light of the recent interest in a cooperative relationship between indigenous healers and representatives of cosmopolitan medicine, to note that the solutions provided by these therapists may tend to deflect attention from recognizing that the problems of their clients often emanate from the stratified and racist nature of American society.

Buxton, M. E., Smith, D. E., and Seymour, R. B. (1987). Spirituality and other points of resistance to the 12-step recovery process. *Journal of Psychoactive Drugs* 19(3):275–286.

De Rios, M. D., and Smith, D. E. (1977). The function of drug rituals in human society: continuities and changes. *Journal of Psychedelic Drugs* 9(3):269–275.

The authors suggest that participation in rituals can be healing and create a positive self image and a feeling of belonging. They also suggest that drug taking in an organized, controlled, and ritualistic manner can have positive effects and need not be addictive or lead to social dysfunctioning.

Roman, Y. M. (1977). Rites of passage: a ritual of detoxification. In *A Multicultural View of Drug Abuse—Proceedings of the National Drug Abuse Conference*, ed. D. E. Smith, S. M. Anderson, M. Buxton, et al., pp. 350–358. Boston: Schenkman.

The author proposes a program directed especially toward a group of heroin (and other illegal substance) abusers who may respond to a directed ritualistic pattern. The addict is taught a self-enhancing ritual that must be performed every day to reinforce a positive identity. The article includes a detailed description of 6 days of ritualistic schedule used in the "rite of passage" therapeutic process.

Singer, M. (1982). Christian Science healing and alcoholism: an anthropological perspective. *Journal of Operational Psychiatry* 13(1):2–12.

The article presents a Christian Science approach to alcoholism therapy that rests upon the concept that Christian Science "denies the existence of matter, sin, death and sickness, and asserts that all is mind, God, and good (p. 2). Christian Science does not deny that people get drunk but rather that this is not caused by alcohol per se, to which only a placebo effect is attributed, but rather by human beliefs and expectations. The author claims that "CS healing and alcoholism psychotherapy . . . can be seen as reflecting core values of Western society, values that often disguise the structural realities of Western social life. Ironically, the enshrinement of individualism ultimately functions to mask the very stresses . . . that are probably central to the etiology of alcoholism" (p. 10).

Singer, M., and Borrero, M. G. (1984). Indigenous treatment for alcoholism: the case of Puerto Rican Spiritism. *Medical Anthropology* 8(4):246–273.

This article is a comprehensive and detailed description of the therapeutic aspects of spiritism and of a Puerto Rican spiritist center in Hartford, Connecticut to treat alcoholics.

Smith, D. E. (1994). AA recovery and spirituality: an addiction medicine perspective. *Journal of Substance Abuse Treatment* 11(2):111–112.

Zinberg, N. E., Jacobsen, R. C., and Harding, W. M. (1975). Social sanctions and rituals as a basis for drug abuse prevention. *American Journal of Drug and Alcohol Abuse* 2(2):165–182.

This article reports on a study the aims of which were "1) to locate and describe controlled users of marijuana, psychedelics, and opiates; 2) to describe various patterns of controlled use; and 3) to identify factors which assist in the development and maintenance of controlled use" (pp. 166–167).

The study located illicit users who "do not fit the stereotyped view of drug users as deviant, sick, out of control. These controlled users are by and large active participants in the larger culture and hold their drug use at levels which do not seriously interfere with ordinary behavior" (pp. 175–176). These users often used drugs in ritual ways and were influenced by sanctions that tended to prevent abuse.

Through self-imposed rituals and sanctions, users who were active members of the society at large were able to use drugs in a controlled manner. As a result the article concludes by supporting legalization of drug taking, not to promote drug taking but to prevent such controlled drug users from being criminalized and from being stigmatized as social deviants.

Zucker, D. K., Austin, F., Fair, A., and Branchey, L. (1987). Associations between patient religiosity and alcohol attitudes and knowledge in an alcohol treatment program. *International Journal of Addictions* 22(1):47–53.

> Studies carried out in generalized populations have shown inverse relationships between degree of religiosity and attitudes towards drinking, knowledge about alcohol, amount of alcohol consumed, and physical complications of alcohol abuse. Within a population of chronic male alcoholics, we found that the more religious patients had a more anti-alcohol attitude; however, none of the other correlations was statistically significant. Within this population, the least religious patients were more likely to change their attitude toward alcohol and to increase their knowledge of the deleterious effects of alcohol after 4 weeks of treatment on an inpatient rehabilitation unit. [p. 47]

12

Shamans

Emboden, W. A., and DeRios, M. D. (1981). Mayan-Egyptian uses of water lilies (Nymphaceae) in shamanic ritual drug use. In *Folk Medicine and Herbal Healing*, ed. G. G. Meyer, K. Blum, and J. G. Cull, pp. 275–286. Springfield, IL: Charles C Thomas.

Peters, L. G., and Price-Williams, D. (1980). Toward an experiential analysis of shamanism. *American Ethnologist* 7:397–418.

> A comprehensive delineation of the ecstatic states of shamans is developed along the lines of cross-cultural psychiatry. Psychiatric concepts, such as dissociation, role playing and hypnosis, are integrated with the ethnographic literature on spirit possession, soul journey and other forms of shamanic ecstasy in order to shed light upon some old anthropological controversies regarding the psychopathology and authenticity of the shaman's trance. Forty-two cultures, from four different cultural areas, are compared in order to determine a set of experiential and psychological factors that collectively identify what is meant by shamanic ecstasy. Shamanic ecstasy is identified as a specific class of ASC involving a) voluntary control of entrance and duration of trance, b) post-trance memory, and c) transic communicative interplay with spectators. [p. 397]

Prince, R. (1988). Shamans and endorphins: hypothesis for a synthesis. *Curare* 11:57–67.

The following passages were particularly noted:

> Hypnosis analgesia is used today for a variety of procedures . . . and in childbirth. The current explanation as to why hypnosis can produce analgesia is that it is due to "reduction of tension and anxiety, promotion of muscle relaxation, and diversion of attention from the pain stimulus." . . . [p. 57]

> These observations suggest that there are at least two distinct mechanisms that could be implicated in endogenously generated analgesia: a purely psychogenic mechanism that we might call "faith" analgesia associated with hypnosis and possibly the placebo effect, and an endorphin-mediated analgesia of the acupuncture type which might be implicated in some drum-and-dance-type phenomena. . . . [p. 58]

> Shamanic trances 1) are frequently associated with motor activities in the form of dance; and 2) almost universally hitherto unexplained fine tremors accompany nonhypnotic trance phenomena. . . . It is possible that the function of trembling is to act as a kind of "endorphin pump." . . . [p. 60]

> The concept that endorphins are generated in response to severe psychological threat suggests a new hypothesis, the mock hyperstress theory. . . . [p. 61]

> The therapeutic effects of some healing systems that make extensive use of dreams can be better understood in the context of mock hyperstress theory. . . . In these examples, highly personalized threat situations are first presented in dreams and then reenacted with the potential for intensified hormonal stress reactions. . . . The theory may also

have relevance in explaining the therapeutic effects of the many Amerindian therapeutic systems that employ the generation of micropsychoses by psychedelic plants. [p. 62]

Ripinsky-Naxon, M. (1989). Hallucinogens, shamanism, and the cultural process. *Anthropos* 84:219–224.

Tiwari, V. J., Padhye, M. D., and Deshmukh, V. K. (1990). Plant hallucinogens and shaman. *Eastern Anthropologist* 43(4): 371–375.

13
Therapeutic Communities/ Outward Bound

Andresen, A. S., and Waal, H. (1978). *Behandlingskollektiv? Bo og Arbeidsfellesskap som Alternativ til Psykatrisk Institusjon.* [*Therapeutic Collective? Living and Work Fellowship as an Alternative to Psychiatric Institutionalization.*] Oslo: Universitetsforlaget.

Bang, A. T., and Bang, R. A. (1991). Community participation in research and action against alcoholism. *World Health Forum* 12:104–109.

Christie, S. D., and DeBerry, S. T. (1994). Culture and community in the therapeutic community: implications for the treatment of recovering substance misusers. *International Journal of the Addictions* 29(6):803–817.

> This paper critically discusses the conceptualization and structure of the therapeutic community employed for the treatment of substance misuse in America. The predominant American model, the concept-house model, is criticized on the grounds that the therapeutic milieu of these treatment agencies is contaminated by their subordinance to the influences of the larger American society. These influences include: the predominance of the medical model,

the agency as an agent of service delivery, capitalism and inequity, implicit views of human nature, and stratification of social structure. The thesis of this paper is that treatment personnel in therapeutic communities must develop increased sensitivity to the larger cultural factors which influence the construction of the therapeutic community. . . . Treatment personnel must be careful to avoid constructing therapeutic communities which too closely mirror the larger culture. [p. 803]

Eriksson, I. (1987). *Missbruks Karriar och Behandling [A Career of Misuse and Therapy.]* Stockholm: Liber.

Furuholmen, D. (1987). *Boka om Veksthuset—Problemet er ikke aa slutte med heroin. Problemet er aa begynne et nytt liv. [The Book about the Growth House—The problem is not to stop heroin use, the problem is to begin a new life.]* Oslo: J. W. Cappelens Forlag A.S.

Houston, M. K., and Drum, A. (1990). Innovative addiction treatment: a combination of traditional therapy and a wilderness based program. In *ICAA, International Institute on the Prevention and Treatment of Alcoholism*, vol. 2, pp. 89–103. Lausanne, Switzerland: *International Council on Alcohol and Addictions.*

This article describes the collaborative addiction treatment program of the Presbyterian/Saint Luke's Medical Center's Addiction Rehabilitation Unit Division and the Colorado Outward Bound School, which has integrated the experiential/adventure-based paradigm with traditional inpatient and outpatient addiction treatment programs.

> For four days, participants are involved in a series of challenging experiences including initiative games, rock climb-

ing, backpacking, rope crossing, and a solo. . . . [p. 92] The Outward Bound experience has three essential components: a unique physical environment, a unique social environment, and the challenges encountered in learning to cope with both. . . . [p. 93] The course is designed to present the addicts with challenges that are similar to what they will encounter in living a life of sobriety. [p. 99]

LaSalvia, T. A. (1993). Enhancing addiction treatment through psychoeducational groups. *Journal of the Substance Abuse Treatment* 10:439–444.

Sandvig, A. (1991). Ungdom i Graasonen—Om samarbeid mellom frivillige organisasjoner. Skole og Tyrilikollektivet. [Youth in the grey zone—concerning collaboration between voluntary organizations, School(s) and the Tyrili collective.] *NotaBene Rapport Nr.* 91:3.

Sorhaug, H. C. (1984). *Ungdom, Ungdomskultur og Ungdomsarbeid.* [*Youth, Youth Culture and Youth Work.*] Oslo: Arbeidsforskningsinstituttene (manuscript).

Stensrud, A. (1985). *Revansj—Ei Bok om Tyrili Kollektivet.* [*Revenge—A Book about the Tyrili Collective.*] Brumundal, Norway: Fagbokforlaget.

Clients with an addiction disorder generally present with an ego deficit in the area of selfcare. This deficiency manifests itself in an inability to suffer and struggle with day-to-day problem solving. Outpatient addiction treatment today places significant resources in psychotherapy and psychodynamic group therapy often at the expense of teaching basic life skills our clients need to negotiate day-to-day living. To address both issues of ego and life skills deficits, the use of a psychoeducational group is presented.

> This specialized, task-oriented didactic group experience is a necessary component of a comprehensive addiction treatment program. A psychoeducational group in the treatment of addictions can serve as a synthesis for problem-solving skills training used in mental health and the psychodynamic theory of addictive behavior. Cases are presented to illustrate the efficacy of psychoeducational groups. [p. 439]

Stensrud, M. K., and Lushbough, R. S. (1988). The implementation of an occupational therapy program in an alcohol and drug dependency treatment center. Special issue: Treatment and Substance Abuse: Psychosocial Occupational Therapy Approaches. *Occupational Therapy in Mental Health* 8(2):1-15.

Thelander, A. (1979). *Hassela Kollektivet—En Rapport om Vardinnehall och Vardideologi pa ett Hem for Unga Narkomaner.* [*The Hassela Collective—A Report about Value Content and Value Ideology in a Home for Young Narcotic Addicts.*] Stockholm: Prisma.

Tyrili-Kollektivet (1989). *For Harde Livet!* [*It is a Matter of Life or Death.*] Aarsmellding. (Annual Report). Tyrili, Norway: Tyrili-Kollektivet.

Vaglum, P. (1979). *Unge Stoffmisbrukere i et "Terapeutisk Samfunn"—Forlop under og efter behandling. En Klinisk Psykiatrisk undersokelse.* [*Young Drug Abusers in a "Therapeutic Community." Results during and after therapy. A Clinical Psychiatric Investigation.*] Oslo: Universitetsforlaget.

—— (1981). Miljoterapi av unge stoffmisbrukere i Norge. [Environmental therapy for young drug abusers in Norway.] *Tidskrift for den Norske Laegeforening* 14(101):852-855.

Waal, H., Andresen, A. S., and Kaada, A. K. (1981). Kollektiver—Hverdag og virkninga. [Collectives—Daily Process and Effect.] Oslo: Universitetsforlaget.

Yablonsky, L. (1989). *The Therapeutic Community: A Successful Approach for Treating Substance Abusers.* New York: Gardner.

14

Traditional Medicine

Baasher, T. A. (1989). Drug and alcohol problems and the developing world. Special Issue: Psychiatry and the Addictions. *International Review of Psychiatry* 1(1–2):13–16.

Jilek, W. G. (1993). Traditional medicine relevant to psychiatry. In *Treatment of Mental Disorders*, ed. N. Sartorius, G. de Girolamo, G. Andrews, et al., pp. 341–390. WHO. [See section on Native American Therapies.]

Two significant sections of this chapter deal with tradition-based group therapies involving altered states of consciousness and indigenous therapy and prevention of alcohol and drug dependence. The following are passages of particular interest:

> Effective use of suggestion and catharsis are important aspects of traditional psychotherapy. . . . [p. 347]

> Altered states of consciousness (ASC) can be induced by physiological techniques (e.g., rhythmic sensory stimulation)

and by psychological influence (e.g., through individual and collective suggestion operant in a specific situation . . . shifting of consciousness). Hypnotherapy is one of the few examples of the therapeutic use of an ASC in modern medicine. . . . [p. 350]

The psychotherapeutic, psychohygienic, prophylactic and socially adaptive functions of ceremonial group activities involving ASCs in non-Western societies have been attested to by several expert observers. . . . [p. 351]

North American Indian dance ceremonials . . . today successfully aim at the rehabilitation of Amerindian individuals whose sociocultural alienation has led to chronic dysphoria with alcohol and drug abuse and anomie depression. . . . [p. 352]

The success of the peyote cult . . . in the rehabilitation of alcoholics has been confirmed by Prof. K. Menninger and other experts. The observed positive results of the peyote cult with Amerindians dependent on alcohol and opiate drugs have been attributed to the hallucinogenic alkaloids and also to the isoquinoline alkaloids in the peyote cactus. . . . [Yet] the effectiveness of the peyote ritual is primarily due not to the bio- and psychoactive substances in the cactus but to the goal-directed group therapeutic process of the ceremonial. . . . [p. 355]

Comparable results in the rehabilitation of alcohol and drug dependents have been achieved without any psychoactive agents in the revived North American Indian dance ceremonials, notably the Gourd Dance, the Sun Dance, and the Winter Spirit Dance. . . . [p. 356]

The aim of the initiation is to help the candidate establish a healthy new existence without alcohol and drug use, and to build up a new personal and cultural identity. This is achieved in a symbolic process of ritualized death and rebirth. . . . The revived Winter Spirit ceremonial has become a most effective preventive and therapeutic program to combat alcohol and drug dependence among Amerindians in the Pacific Northwest. . . . [p. 356]

The article also includes traditional therapeutic measures used to combat drug addiction in African, Latin American, Buddhist, and Islamic cultures.

Latin American Cultures: Puerto Rican espiritismo healers [and] . . . Mexican folk healers treat alcoholics by counseling, social engineering, symbolic ritual acts, and the administration of herbal sedatives. The use of aversion therapy . . . deconditioning with emetic herbal teas, to be taken together with alcoholic drinks, is practiced in a healing compound of the Colorado Indians of Ecuador, frequented by rural and urban patients. In northern Peru, curanderos also use aversion therapy with herbal emetics and laxatives . . . Chronic alcoholic patients are admitted to a healing compound and undergo a process of emotional and physical fortification.

Buddhist cultures: [The UN is interested in] integrating traditional shamanic ceremonies into modern detoxification and rehabilitation programs.

In Japan, traditional practices of the Shinshu Buddhist sect have been adapted for the rehabilitation of alcoholics in the form of naikan (self-examination therapy), which, complemented by a culture-congenial group approach (danshukai) has become a valuable therapeutic resource in the management of alcohol dependence. . . . [p. 359]

Islamic cultures: The integration of Islamic spiritual approaches in the therapy of drug addiction has been pioneered in Egypt and Saudi Arabia. In 1977, a treatment unit for drug addicts was established at Abu El Azayem Mosque in Cairo, in which the religious leader (sheikh) assumed special functions in the therapeutic team by holding group meetings providing religious teaching with emphasis on Islamic injunctions regarding dependence-producing substance use, encouraging the strengthening of social ties. . . . The addiction unit at Shahar Hospital, Taif, Saudi Arabia, has for several years now integrated a program of religious therapy in which the mosque is the center of therapeutic activity; 75% of problems with "inner religious considerations" maintained abstinence over 2 years, as compared to 33% of problems motivated by other considerations.

Black-African religious movements: Independent Black African churches of South Africa (Zionist, Ethiopian, Apostolic). . . . Members are subject to proscriptions which usually include an injunction against the consumption of alcoholic beverages and in many cases against the use of drugs.

Counseling is conducted by faith healers and former alcoholic church members; often there is also dream interpretation by authorized leaders. . . . [p. 361]

Summary:

1) In general, tradition-based practices provide effective therapeutic management for neurotic disorders (especially with dissociation and conversion symptoms), for psychosomatic and somatoform disorders, for psychosocial problems, and for reactive depressions, including self-destructive behavior.

2) Traditional medicine practices, ritual procedures and sedative herbal remedies are effective in treatment of reactive and transient psychoses and psychosis-like, culture-bound syndromes.

3) In the treatment, rehabilitation, and prevention of alcohol and drug dependence, therapeutic practices based

> on indigenous cultural and religious traditions have, in many instances, been as successful and sometimes more successful than "official" treatment and rehabilitation programs. [p. 363]

Spencer, C. P., Heggenhougen, H. K., and Navaratnam, V. (1980). Traditional therapies and the treatment of drug dependence in Southeast Asia. *American Journal of Chinese Medicine* 8(3):230–238.

Suwaki, H. (1979). "Naikan" and "Danshukai" for the treatment of Japanese alcoholic patients. *British Journal of the Addictions* 74:15–19.

> The author describes two important therapies, Naikan Therapy and Danshukai, in treating Japanese alcoholics. Naikan therapy is a method which is administered mainly in hospitals and is most suitable for patients to reflect on their past lives, retrieve the bonds of affection of their families and make up their minds to abstain from alcohol. Danshukai is an important method, particularly as after-care following discharge in the sense that patients continue sticking to the resolution to give up drinking they made in the hospital, while keeping in touch with their fellow members for encouragement. These two methods were born in the Japanese Buddhist climate and are much alike in their basic principles. Particularly, regarding the family as important and making efforts with the family are outstanding features common to these two methods, and they can be administered one after the other to provide a synthetical effect. [p. 15]

Trotter, R. T. (1979). Evidence of an ethnomedical form of aversion therapy on the United States-Mexico border. *Journal of Ethnopharmacology* 1:279–284.

Ethnographic data are presented on the use of a seed, haba de San Ignacio (Hura polyandra L. and Hura crepitans L), indicating its ability to inhibit Mexican-American problem drinkers from imbibing alcohol. The seed is most often administered by a family member without the knowledge of the abusive drinker her/himself, thus ruling out a psychosomatic or placebo effect.

References

Agar, M. (1973). *Ripping and Running: A Formal Ethnography of Urban Heroin Addicts.* New York: Seminar Press.
—— (1975). *Into that whole thing: ritualistic drug use among urban American drug addicts.* Paper presented at the Society of Applied Anthropology, Amsterdam, September.
Albaugh, B. J., and Anderson, P. O. (1974). Peyote in the treatment of alcoholism among American Indians. *American Journal of Psychiatry* 131(11):1247–1250.
Allen, J. W., and Merlin, M. D. (1992). Psychoactive mushroom use in Koh Samui and Koh Pha-Ngan, Thailand. *Journal of Ethnopharmacology* 35:205–228.
Anderson, D. (1977). Transcendental meditation as an alternative to heroin abuse in service. *American Journal of Psychiatry* 134(11):1308–1309.
Andresen, A. S., and Waal, H. (1978). *Behandlingskollektiv? Bo og Arbeidsfellesskap som Alternativ til Psykatrisk Institusjon.* [*Therapeutic Collective? Living and Work Fellowship as an Alternative to Psychiatric Institution(alization).*] Oslo: Universitetsforlaget.
Arokiasamy, C. M. V., and Taricone, P. T. (1992). Drug rehabilitation in West Malaysia: an overview of its history and development. *International Journal of the Addictions* 27(11): 1301–1311.

References

Arredondo, R., Weddige, R. L., Justice, C. L., and Fitz, J. (1987). Alcoholism in Mexican-Americans: intervention and treatment. *Hospital and Community Psychiatry* 38(2):180–183.

Baasher, T. A., ed. Traditional psychotherapeutic practices in the Sudan. Unpublished manuscript.

Baasher, T. A., and Abn el Azayem, G. M. (1980). Egypt: the role of the mosque in treatment. In *Drug Problems in Sociocultural Context—A Basis for Policies and Programme Planning*. ed. G. Edwards and A. Arif, Public Health Papers No. 73, pp. 131–134. Geneva: WHO.

Baer, H. A. (1981). Prophets and advisors in black spiritual churches: Therapy, palliative, or opiate? *Culture, Medicine, and Psychiatry* 5:145–170.

Bang, A. T., and Bang, R. A. (1991). Community participation in research and action against alcoholism. *World Health Forum* 12:104–109.

Belfer, M., and Heggenhougen, H. K. (1995). Substance abuse. In *World Mental Health*, ed. R. Desjarlais, L. Eisenberg, B. Good, et al., pp. 87–115. Oxford: Oxford University Press.

Benson, H. (1969). Yoga for drug abuse. *New England Journal of Medicine* 281:1133.

Benson, H., and Wallace, R. K. (1972). Decreased drug abuse with transcendental meditation—a study of 1,862 subjects. In *Drug Abuse: Proceedings of the International Conference*, ed. C. J. D. Zarafantis, pp. 369–376. Philadelphia: Lea & Febiger.

Bergman, R. L. (1971). Navajo peyote use: its apparent safety. *American Journal of Psychiatry* 128(6):51–55.

Blum, K., Futternman, S. L., and Pascarosa, P. (1977). Peyote, a potential ethnopharmacologic agent for alcoholism and other drug dependencies: possible biochemical rationale. *Clinical Toxicology* 11(4):459–472.

Blum, K., and Tilton, J. E. (1981). Understanding the high mind. In *Folk Medicine and Herbal Healing*, ed. G. G. Meyer, K. Blum, and J. G. Cull, pp. 261–274. Springfield, IL: Charles C Thomas.

Bourguignon, E. (1973). *Religion, Altered States of Consciousness and Social Change*. Athens, OH: Ohio University Press.

—— (1977). Altered states of consciousness, myths, and rituals. In *Drugs, Rituals and Altered States of Consciousness*, ed. B. M. DuToit, pp. 7–23. Rotterdam: A. A. Balkema.

Bourne, P. G. (1975). Non pharmacological approaches to the treatment of drug abuse. *American Journal of Chinese Medicine* 3(3):235–244.

Bowers, J. Z., and Carruba, R. W. (1978). Drug abuse and sexual binding spells in seventeenth century Asia: essays from the Amoenitatum Exoticarum of Engelbert Kaempfer. *Journal of Historical Medicine and Allied Sciences* 33(3):318–343.

Brinkman, D. N. (1978). Biofeedback application to drug addiction in the University of Colorado drug rehabilitation program. *International Journal of the Addictions* 13(5):817–830.

Brown, B. (1975). Biofeedback: an exercise in "self-control." *Saturday Review*, Feb. 22, pp. 22–26.

Brown, J. K., and Malone, M. H. (1975). Legal highs:—constituents, activity, toxicology and herbal folklore. *Clinic Toxicology* 12(1):1–31.

Brown, K. L. (1984). Hallucinogenic mushrooms, jade, obsidian, and the Guatemalan Highlands: what did the Olmecs really want? In *Trade and Exchange in Early Mesoamerica*, ed. K. G. Hirth, pp. 215–233. Albuquerque: University of New Mexico Press.

Brumbaugh, A. G. (1993). Acupuncture: new perspectives in chemical dependency treatment. *Journal of Substance Abuse Treatment* 10:35–43.

Bullock, M. L., Culliton, P. D., and Olander, R. T. (1989). Controlled trial of acupuncture for severe recidivist alcoholism. *Lancet* 1(8652):1435–1439.

Burkill, I. H. (1966). *A Dictionary of the Economic Products of the Malay Peninsula*, vols. 1 and 2, 2nd ed. Kuala Lumpur: Ministry of Agriculture and Co-operatives.

Burkill, I. H., and Haniff, M. (1930). Malay village medicine, The Gardens' Bulletin. *Straits Settlements* 6(2):167–332.

Buxton, M. E., Smith, D. E., and Seymour, R. B. (1987). Spirituality and other points of resistance to the 12-step recovery process. *Journal of Psychoactive Drugs* 19(3):275–286.

Cappendijk, S. L. T., and Dzoljic, M. R. (1993). Inhibitory effects of ibogaine on cocaine self-administration in rats. *European Journal of Pharmacology* 241:261–265.

Chandrasena, R. (n.d.). Opium dependence following treatment—Traditional practitioners in Sri Lanka. Unpublished manuscript.

Chen, J. Y. P. (1972). Acupuncture. In *Medicine and Public Health in the People's Republic of China*, DHEW (NIH) Publ. No. 72-67, ed. J. R. Quinn, pp. 65–90. Washington, DC: J. E. Fogarty International Center.

Chen, P. C. Y. (1970a). Indigenous concepts of causation and methods of prevention of childhood diseases in a rural Malay community. *Journal of Tropical Pediatrics* 16:33–42.

—— (1970b). Indigenous Malay psychotherapy. *Tropical and Geographical Medicine* 22:409–415.

—— (1973). Indigenous Malay surgery. *Tropical and Geographical Medicine* 25:95–99.

—— (1975). Medical systems in Malaysia: culture bases and differential use. *Social Science and Medicine* 9:171–180.

—— (1981). Traditional and modern medicine in Malaysia. *Social Science and Medicine* 15A:127–136.

Christie, S. D., and DeBerry, S. T. (1994). Culture and community in the therapeutic community: implications for the treatment of recovering substance misusers. *International Journal of the Addictions* 29(6):803–817.

Clement-Jones, V., Lowry, P. J., McLoughlin, L., et al. (1979). Acupuncture in heroin addicts: changes in met-enkephalin and beta-endorphin in blood and cerebrospinal fluid. *Lancet* 2(8139):380–382.

Clements, G., Krenner, L., and Molk, W. (1988). The use of the transcendental meditation programme in the prevention of drug abuse and in the treatment of drug-addicted persons. *Bulletin on Narcotics* 40(1):51–56.

Colley, F. C. (1978). Traditional Indian medicine in Malaysia. *Journal of the Malaysian British Royal Asiatic Society* 51(part 1):77–109.

Collins, J. M. (1950). The Indian Shaker Church: a study of continuity and change in religion. *Southwestern Journal of Anthropology* 6:399–411.

Colson, A. C. (1971). The differential use of medical resources in developing countries. *Journal of Health and Social Behavior* 12:226–237.

Corcoran, J. P., and Longo, E. D. (1992). Psychological treatment of anabolic-androgenic steroid-dependent individuals. *Journal of Substance Abuse Treatment* 9:229–235.

Cowley, G., Heiman, H., and Ramo, J. C. (1993). A psychedelic trip to the end of addiction. *Newsweek*, August 23, p. 45.

Crawford, R. J. M. (1989). Follow up of alcohol and other drug dependents treated with psychodrama. *New Zealand Medical Journal* 102(866):199.

Davis, W. (1985). Hallucinogenic plants and their use in traditional societies—an overview. *Cultural Survival Quarterly* 9(4):2–5.

Deecher, D. C., Teitler, M., Soderlund, D. M., et al. (1992). Mechanisms of action of ibogaine and harmaline congeners based on radioligand binding studies. *Brain Research* 571:242–247.

Deitch, D., and Solit, R. (1993). International training for drug abuse treatment and the issue of cultural relevance. *Journal of Psychoactive Drugs* 25(1):87–95.

Denney, M. R., Baugh, J. L., and Hardt, H. D. (1991). Sobriety outcome after alcoholism treatment with biofeedback participation: a pilot inpatient study. *International Journal of the Addictions* 26(3):335–341.

DeRios, M. D. (1986). Enigma of drug-induced altered states of consciousness among the !Kung Bushmen of the Kalahari Desert. *Journal of Ethnopharmacology* 15:297–304.

DeRios, M. D., and Smith, D. E. (1977). The function of drug rituals in human society: continuities and changes. *Journal of Psychedelic Drugs* 9(3):269–275.

—— (1984). Drug use and abuse in cross-cultural perspective. In *Culture and Psychopathology*, ed. J. E. Mezzich and C. E. Berganza, pp. 385–399. New York: Columbia University Press.

deSilva, P. (1983). The Buddhist attitude to alcoholism. In *Drug Use and Misuse—Cultural Perspectives (Based on a Collaborative Study by the World Health Organization)*, ed. G. Edwards, A. Arif, and J. Jaffe, pp. 33–41. London: Croom Helm.

Dunn, F. L. (1974). Traditional beliefs and practices affecting medical care in Malaysian Chinese communities. *Medical Journal of Malaysia* 29(1):7–10.

—— (1975). Medical care in the Chinese community in Peninsular Malaysia. In *Medicine in Chinese Cultures: Comparative Studies on Health Care in Chinese and Other Societies*, ed. A. Kleinman, et al. DHEW Publ. No. NIH 75-683, pp. 297–326. Washington, DC: U. S. Dept. of Health, Education, and Welfare.

—— (1976). Traditional Asian medicine and cosmopolitan medicine as adaptive systems. In *Asian Medical Systems*, ed. C. Leslie, pp. 133–158. Berkeley: University of California Press.

Dushman, R. D., and Bressler, M. J. (1991). Psychodrama in an adolescent chemical dependency treatment program. *Individual Psychology* 47(4):515–520.

DuToit, B. M. (1977a). *Drugs, Rituals and Altered States of Consciousness*. Rotterdam: A. A. Balkema.

——— (1977b). Introduction. In *Drugs, Rituals and Altered States of Consciousness*, pp. 1–4. Rotterdam: A. A. Balkema.

Edwards, G. (1983). Countries differ in their treatment of drug problems. In *Drug Use and Misuse—Cultural Perspectives (Based on a Collaborative Study by the World Health Organization)*, ed. G. Edwards, A. Arif, and J. Jaffe, pp. 176–184. London: Croom Helm.

Edwards, G., and Arif, A. (1983). The future. In *Drug Use and Misuse—Cultural Perspectives (Based on a Collaborative Study by the World Health Organization)*, ed. G. Edwards, A. Arif, and J. Jaffe, pp. 269–274. London: Croom Helm.

Edwards, G., Arif, A., and Jaffe, J., eds. (1983). *Drug Use and Misuse—Cultural Perspectives (Based on a Collaborative Study by the World Health Organization)*. London: Croom Helm.

Emboden, W. A. (1972). *Narcotic Plants*. New York: Macmillan.

Emboden, W. A., and DeRios, M. D. (1981). Mayan-Egyptian uses of water lilies (Nymphaceae) in shamanic ritual drug use. In *Folk Medicine and Herbal Healing*, ed. G. G. Meyer, K. Blum, and J. G. Cull, pp. 275–286. Springfield, IL: Charles C Thomas.

Engelmajer, L. J. (1985). *Le Patnarche—pour les Drogues: l. Espoir.* France: Le Patre.

Equinox Group (1988). The equinox system and heroin addiction—mechanisms implicated in the application of acupuncture, electroacupuncture and electrostimulation for drug withdrawal. *Equinox Review* 4:1–4.

Eriksson, I. (1987). *Missbruks Karriar och Behandling.* [*A Career of Misuse and Therapy.*] Stockholm: Liber.

Fernandez, J. W. (1972). Tabernanthe Iboga: narcotic ecstasies and the work of the ancestors. In *Flesh of the Gods—The Ritual Use of Hallucinogens*, ed. P. T. Furst, pp. 237–260. New York: Praeger.

Frye, R. V. (1990). Affective modes in multimodality addiction treatment. In *Treatment Choices for Alcoholism and Substance Abuse*, ed. H. B. Milkman and L. I. Sederer, pp. 287–307. Lexington, MA: Lexington Books.

Furst, P. T. (1972). To find our life: peyote among the Hichol Indians of Mexico. In *Flesh of the Gods—The Ritual Use of Hallucinogens*, ed. P. T. Furst, pp. 36–184. New York: Praeger.

—— (1976). *Hallucinogens and Culture*. San Francisco: Chandler and Sharpe.

——, ed. (1972). *Flesh of the Gods—The Ritual Use of Hallucinogens*. New York: Praeger.

Furuholmen, D. (1987). *Boka om Veksthuset—Problemet er Ikke aa Slutte Med Heroin. Problemet er aa Begynne et Nytt Liv.* [*The Book about the Veksthus (Growth House): The problem is not to stop heroin use, the problem is to begin a new life.*] Oslo: J. W. Cappelens Forlag A.S.

Galanter, M., and Buckley, P. (1978). Evangelical religion and meditation: psychotherapeutic effects. *Journal of Nervous and Mental Disease* 166(10):685–691.

Galanter, M., Rabking, R., et al. (1979). The "Moonies": a psychological study of the conversion and membership on a contemporary religious sect. *American Journal of Psychiatry* 136(2):165–170.

Ganguli, H. C. (1985). Meditation subculture and drug use. *Human Relations* 38(10):953–962.

Gelderloos, P., Walton, K. G., Orme-Johnson, D. W., and Alexander, C. N. (1991). Effectiveness of the transcendental meditation program in preventing and treating substance misuse: a review. *International Journal of the Addictions* 26(3):293–325.

Giannini, A. J., Miller, N. S., and Turner, C. E. (1992). Treatment of Khat addiction. *Journal of Substance Abuse Treatment* 9:379–382.

Gimlette, J. D. (1915). *Malay Poisons and Charm Cures*. Kuala Lumpur: Oxford University Press, 1975.

Gimlette, J. D., and Burkill, I. H. (1930). *The Medical Book of Malayan Medicine, The Gardens' Bulletin*, S. S., vol. vi, April.

Gimlette, J. D., and Thomson, H. W. (1939). *A Dictionary of Malayan Medicine*. Oxford: Oxford University Press.

Glick, S. D., Gallagher, C. A., Hough, L. B., et al. (1992). Differential effects of ibogaine pretreatment on brain levels of morphine and (+)amphetamine. *Brain Research* 588:173–176.

Glick, S. D., Rossman, K., Steindorf, S., et al. (1991). Effects and aftereffects of ibogaine on morphine self-administration in rats. *European Journal of Pharmacology* 195:341–345.

Greve, J., ed. (1993). *Norway—A Leading Country in Rehabilitation of People with Disabilities* (Focus on the Potential 1993), Organizing Committee for the Expert Meeting: Focus on the Potential. Norway: Fagernes.

Hamarneh, S. (1972). Pharmacy in medieval Islam and the history of drug addiction. *Medical History* 16(3):226–237.

Hare, H. A., Caspari, C., Rusby, H. H., et al. (1909). *The National Standard Dispensatory*. Philadelphia: Lea and Febiger.

Harner, M. J. (1973). *Hallucinogens and Shamanism*. New York: Oxford University Press.

Heggenhougen, H. K. (1979). Meeting of Malaysia traditional healers. *Medical Anthropology Newsletter* 11:3.

—— (1980a). The utilization of traditional medicine—a Malaysian example. *Social Science and Medicine* 14B:39–44.

—— (1980b). Bomohs, doctors and sinsehs—medical pluralisms in Malaysia. *Social Science and Medicine* 14B:235–244.

—— (1984). Traditional medicine and treatment of drug addicts—

three examples from Southeast Asia. *Medical Anthropology Quarterly* 16(1):3-7.

—— (1985). Pain, addiction and traditional therapy in Southeast Asia. *Social History of Medicine Bulletin* 36:16-17.

Heggenhougen, H. K., and Navaratnam, V. (1979a). Traditional therapies in drug dependence management, excerpts used for Herbal therapy in the war on drug addiction. *UNESCO Courier*, July, pp. 38-39.

—— (1979b). *A General Overview on the Practices Relating to the Traditional Treatment of Drug Dependents in Malaysia.* Siri Monograph. Penang, Malaysia: National Drug Dependence Research Centre.

Higgins, S. T., Delancy, D. D., Budney, A. J., et al. (1991). A behavioral approach to achieving initial cocaine abstinence. *American Journal of Psychiatry* 148(9):1218-1224.

Hill, T. W. (1990). Peyotism and the control of heavy drinking: the Nebraska Winnebago in the early 1900s. *Human Organization* 49(3):255-265.

Hopson, J. L. (1988). A pleasurable chemistry. *Psychology Today*, July/August, pp. 29-33.

Houston, M. K., and Drum, A. (1990). Innovative addiction treatment: a combination of traditional therapy and a wilderness-based program. In ICAA, *31st International Institute on the Prevention and Treatment of Alcoholism*. Proceedings, vol. 2, ed. E. Tongue and A. Tongue, pp. 89-103. Rome, Italy, 1985.

Howard, J. H. (1976). The Plains gourd dance as a revitalization movement. *American Ethnologist* 3:243-259.

Ja, D. Y., and Aoki, B. (1993). Substance abuse treatment: cultural barriers in the Asian-American community. *Journal of Psychoactive Drugs* 25(1):61-71.

Jaffee, J. H. (1977). Some reflections on the evolution of current American approaches to problems of drug abuse and to the treatment of drug abusers. *Journal of Drug Issues* 7(1):1-12.

Jetter, A. (1994). The psychedelic cure. *The New York Times Magazine*, April 10, 50–52.

Jilek, W. G. (1978). Native renaissance: the survival and revival of indigenous therapeutic ceremonials among North American Indians. *Transcultural Psychiatric Research* 15:117–147.

—— (1989). Therapeutic use of altered states of consciousness in contemporary North American Indian dance ceremonials. In *Altered States of Consciousness and Mental Health— A Cross-Cultural Perspective*. Cross Cultural Research and Methodology series, vol. 12, ed. C. A. Ward, pp. 167–185. Newbury Park, CA: Sage.

—— (1992). The renaissance of shamanic dance in Indian populations of North America. *Diogenes* (Summer) 158:87–100.

—— (1993a). Traditional medicine relevant to psychiatry. In *Treatment of Mental Disorders*, ed. N. Sartorius, G. de Girolamo, G. Andrews, et al., pp. 341–390. Geneva, Switzerland: WHO.

—— (1993b). Traditional healing against alcoholism and drug dependence. *Curare* 17:145–160.

Jilek-Aall, L., and Jilek, W. G. (1985). Buddhist temple treatment of narcotic addiction and neurotic-psychosomatic disorders in Thailand. In *Psychiatry: The State of the Art*, vol. 8, ed. P. P. P. Berner, R. Wolf, et al., pp. 673–677. New York: Plenum.

Johnson, L. (1990). Creative therapies in the treatment of addictions: the art of transforming shame. *The Arts in Psychotherapy* 17:2750–2755.

Johnson, R. E., Jaffe, R. H., and Fudala, P. P. J. (1992). A controlled trial of buprenoriphne treatment for opioid dependence. *Journal of the American Medical Association* 267(20): 27S–55.

Johnson, S. H. (1983). Treatment of drug abusers in Malaysia: a comparison. *International Journal of the Addictions* 18(7): 951–958.

Jonas, D. F., and Jonas, A. D. (1977). A bioanthropological overview of addiction. *Perspectives in Biology and Medicine* 20:345–354.

Kao, A. A., and Lu, L. Y. C. (1974). Acupuncture procedure for treating drug addiction. *American Journal of Acupuncture* 2(3):201–207.

Khant, U. (1985). Measures to prevent and reduce drug abuse among young people in Burma. *Bulletin on Narcotics* 37(2, 3): 81–89.

King, G. (1992). Gardenia King. *Mother Jones*, January/February, p. 47.

Klajner, F., Hartman, L. M., and Sobell, M. B. (1984). Treatment of substance abuse by relaxation training: a review of its rationale, efficacy and mechanisms. *Addictive Behaviors* 9:41–55.

Kurland, A. A., Unger, S., Shaffer, J. W., and Savage, C. (1967). Psychedelic therapy utilizing LSD in the treatment of the alcoholic patient: a preliminary report. *American Journal of Psychiatry* 123(10):1202–1209.

LaBarre, W. (1972). Hallucinogens and the shamanic origins of religion. In *Flesh of the Gods*, ed. P. T. Furst, pp. 261–278. New York: Praeger.

—— (1975). Anthropological perspectives on hallucination and hallucinogens. In *Behavior, Experience and Theory*, ed. R. K. Siegal and L. J. West, pp. 9–52. New York: Wiley.

—— (1977). Anthropological views of cannabis. *Reviews in Anthropology* A(3):237–250.

Lamontagne, Y., Hand, I., Annable, L., and Gagnon, M.-A. (1975). Physiological and psychological effects of alpha and EMG feedback training with college drug users. A pilot study. *Canadian Psychiatric Association Journal* 20(5):337–348.

LaSalvia, T. A. (1993). Enhancing addiction treatment through psychoeducational groups. *Journal of Substance Abuse Treatment* 10:439–444.

Lau, M. P. (1976). Acupuncture and addiction: an overview. *Addictive Diseases: an International Journal* 2(3):449–463.

Lee, R. L. M. (1985). Alternative systems in Malaysian drug rehabilitation: organization and control in comparative perspective. *Social Science and Medicine* 21(11):1289–1296.

——— (1989). Self-presentation in Malaysian spirit scances: a dramaturgical perspective on altered states of consciousness in healing ceremonies. In *Altered States of Consciousness and Mental Health—A Cross-Cultural Perspective*, ed. C. A. Ward, Cross-Cultural Research and Methodology Series, vol. 12, pp. 251–266. Newbury Park, CA: Sage.

Lemlij, M. (1978). Primitive group treatment. *Psychiatric Clinics* 11:10–14.

Lex, B. (1975). Physiological aspects of ritual trance. *Journal of Altered States of Consciousness* 2.

——— (1987). Review of alcohol problems in ethnic minority groups. *Journal of Consulting and Clinical Psychology* 55(3): 293–300.

Lex, B., and Meyer, R. (1977). Opiate receptors and opiate antagonists: progress in the "war on drugs." *Journal of Drug Issues* 7(1):54–60.

Lex, B., and Schor, N. (1977). A proposed bioanthropological approach linking ritual and opiate addiction. *Addictive Diseases* 3(2):287–303.

Lowinger, P. (1977). The solution to narcotic addiction in the People's Republic of China. *American Journal of Drug and Alcohol Abuse* 4(2):165–178.

Lugman, W. F., and Danowski, T. (1976). The use of khat (Catha edulis) in Yemen. Social and medical observations. *Annals of Internal Medicine* 85(2):246–249.

Mahony, J., and Waller, D. (1992). Art therapy in the treatment of alcohol and drug abuse. In *Art Therapy: A Handbook*, ed. D. Waller and A. Gilroy, pp. 173–188. Buckingham: Open University Press.

Maisonneuve, I. M., and Glick, S. D. (1992). Interactions between ibogaine and cocaine in rats: in vivo microdialysis and motor behavior. *European Journal of Pharmacology* 212: 263–266.

Mala, T. A. (1985). Alcoholism and mental health treatment in circumpolar areas: traditional and non-traditional approaches. *Circumpolar Health* 84:332–334.

Margolin, A., Change, P., Avants, S. K., and Kosten, T. R. (1993). Effects of sham and real auricular needling: implications for trials of acupuncture for cocaine addiction. *American Journal of Chinese Medicine* 21(2):103–111.

Martin, R. T. (1970). The role of coca in the history, religion and medicine of South American Indians. *Economic Botany* 24:422.

Marx, J. L. (1975). Opiate receptors—implications and applications. *Science* 189:708–710.

McBride, C. A. (1910). *The Modern Treatment of Alcoholism and Drug Narcotism*. London: London Press.

McCoy, A. (1972). *The Politics of Heroin in Southeast Asia*. New York: Harper & Row.

McDonald, D. (1990). Ayurveda and acupuncture in heroin detoxification in Sri Lanka. *Drug and Alcohol Review* 9:329–331.

McDonald, E. (1985). Creative writing therapy used to assist chemically dependent adolescents express feelings. In *ICAA, Alcohol, Drugs and Tobacco*, pp. 130–132. Lausanne: ICAA.

McGovern, M. P. (1982). Alcoholism in Southeast Asia—prevalence and treatment. *International Journal of Psychiatry* 28:36–44.

McKay, D. A. (1971). Food, illness and folk medicine: insights from Ulu Trengganu, West Malaysia. *Ecology of Food and Nutrition* 1:67–72.

McLelland, A. T., Grissom, G. R., Brill, P. P., et al. (1993). Private substance abuse treatments: are some programs more effective than others? *Journal of Substance Abuse Treatment* 10:243–254.

McLelland, A. T., Grossman, D. S., Blaine, J. D., and Haverkos, H. W. (1993). Acupuncture treatment for drug abuse: a technical review. *Journal of Substance Abuse Treatment* 10:569–576.

McPeake, J. D., Kennedy, B. P., and Gordon, S. M. (1991). Altered states of consciousness therapy—a missing component in alcohol and drug rehabilitation treatment. *Journal of Substance Abuse Treatment* 8:75–82.

Meltes, J. (1977). The 1977 Nobel prize in physiology or medicine. *Science* 198:594–596.

Miller, W. R. (1992). The effectiveness of treatment of substance abuse. *Journal of Substance Abuse Treatment* 9:93–102.

Mohd. Taib Osman (1972). Patterns of supernatural premises underlying the institution of the bomoh in Malay culture. *Bijdragen tot de Taal. Landen Volkekunde* 128:219–234.

—— (1976). The bomoh and the practice of Malay medicine. *South East Asia Review* 1(1):16–26.

Morinis, E. A. (1978). Two pathways in understanding disease: traditional and scientific. *WHO Chronicle* 32:57–60.

NADA (National Acupuncture Detoxification Association) (1990). *Nada Pamphlet*, p. 4. New York: NADA.

Nathan, R. G., Robinson, D., Cherek, D. R., et al. (1986). Alternative treatments for withdrawing the long-term benzodiazepine user: a pilot study. *International Journal of the Addictions* 21(2):195–211.

Nebelkopf, E. (1987). Herbal therapy in the treatment of drug use. *International Journal of the Addictions* 22(8):695–717.

—— (1988). Herbs and substance abuse treatment: a 10-year perspective. *Psychoactive Drugs* 20(3):349–354.

Negrete, J. C. (1978). Coca leaf chewing: a public health assessment. *European Journal of Addiction* 73:289–290.

Neher, A. (1962). A physiological explanation of unusual behaviours in ceremonies involving drums. *Human Biology* 34:151–161.

Nelson, G. R. (1975). The psychology of hypnotic drug detoxifications. *Journal of the American Society of Psychosomatic Dentistry and Medicine* 22(2):44–50.

Newmeyer, J. A., Johnson, G., and Klot, S. (1984). Acupuncture as a detoxification modality. *Journal of Psychoactive Drugs* 16(3):241–261.

Newmeyer, J. A., and Whitehead, C. (1977). Acupuncture and heroin addiction: a summary of the experience of the Haight-Ashbury Free Medical Clinic. In *A Multicultural View of Drug Abuse—Proceedings of the National Drug Abuse Conference*, ed. D. E. Smith, S. M. Anderson, M. Buxton, et al., pp. 404–409. Boston: Schenkman.

Pardeck, J. T. (1991). Using books to prevent and treat adolescent chemical dependency. *Adolescence* 26(101):201–208.

Pascarosa, P., and Futterman, S. (1976). Ethnopsychedelic therapy for alcoholics: observations in the peyote ritual of the Native American Church. *Journal of Psychedelic Drugs* 8(3):215–221.

Patterson, M. A. (1974). Electro-acupuncture in alcoholism and drug addictions. *Clinical Medicine* 81:9–13.

—— (1975). *Addictions Can Be Cured—The Treatment of Drug Addiction by Neuro-Electric Stimulation.* Berhamsted, Herts., UK: Lion.

—— (1976). Effects of neuro-electric therapy (NET) in drug addiction: interim report. *Bulletin on Narcotics* 28(4):55–62.

—— (1977). *A new approach to treatment.* Paper for a European Symposium for Christians Caring for Those Involved in Addiction and Allied Social Problems.

——— (1993). Neuroelectric therapy (NET) in addictions. *Neuroelectric Therapy*, pp. 1–4. Manuscript. Glasgow: NET.
Patterson, M. A., Patterson, L., Flood, N. V., et al. (1993). Electrostimulation in drug and alcohol detoxification—significance of stimulation criteria in clinical success. *Addiction Research* 1:13–44.
Pelletier, K. R. (1977). *Mind as Healer. Mind as Slayer*. New York: Dell.
Peters, L. G., and Price-Williams, D. (1980). Toward an experiential analysis of shamanism. *American Ethnologist* 7:397–418.
Petersen, R. C. (1977). History of cocaine. In *Cocaine*, ed. R. C. Petersen and R. C. Stillman. NIDA Research Monograph No. 13. Washington, DC: DHEW.
Pigot, R. (1975). The concept of altered states of consciousness and how it helps us understand the drug scene. *Medical Journal of Australia* 2(23):882–884.
Poshyachinda, V. (1980). Thailand: treatment at the Tam Kraborg Temple. In *Drug Problems in Sociocultural Context—A Basis for Policies and Programme Planning*, ed. G. Edwards and A. Arif, Public Health Papers No. 73, pp. 121–125. Geneva: WHO.
——— (1982). *Indigenous drug dependence treatment in Thailand.* Paper presented at the 7th meeting of ASEAN drug experts, Pattaya, Thailand, November/December.
——— (1984). Indigenous treatment for drug dependence in Thailand. *Impact of Science on Society* 34(1):67–76.
——— (1993). *A review on the Buddhist temple drug dependence treatment in Thailand.* Paper presented at the meeting of WHO Substance Abuse Collaborating Centres, Geneva, September.
Poshyachinda, V., et al. (1978). *Evaluation of Treatment Outcome—The Buddhist Temple Treatment Center, Tam Kraborg*. Bangkok: Institute of Health Research, Chulalongkorn University.

Prabhakaran, L. G. (1979). *The pharmacological examination and characterization of natural products and preparations used in drug detoxification.* Thesis, School of Pharmaceutical Sciences, University Sains Malaysia, Penang.

Preeja, P. (1978). Personal communication, from field notes. October, Thailand.

Prince, R. (1988). Shamans and endorphins: hypothesis for a synthesis. *Curare* 11:57–67.

Quinn, J. R., ed. (1972). *Medicine and Public Health in the People's Republic of China.* DHEW (NIH) Publ. No. 72-67. Washington, DC: J. E. Fogarty International Center.

—— (1974). *China Medicine As We Saw It.* DHEW Publ. No. (NIH) 75-684. Washington, DC: J. E. Fogarty International Center.

Richards, L. G. (1979). Personal communication. (Division of Research, NIDA, Rockville, Maryland, USA.)

Ridley, H. N. (1906). Malay drugs. *Agricultural Bulletin of the Straits and the Federated Malay States* 5(6, 7), 8(6).

Riet, G. T., Kleijnen, J., and Knipschild, P. (1990). A meta-analysis of studies into the effect of acupuncture on addiction. *British Journal of General Practice* 40(338):379–382.

Ripinsky-Naxon, M. (1989). Hallucinogens, shaminism, and the cultural process. *Anthropos* 84:219–224.

Roman, Y. M. (1977). Rites of passage: a ritual of detoxification. In *A Multicultural View of Drug Abuse—Proceedings of the National Drug Abuse Conference, 1977,* ed. D. E. Smith, S. M. Anderson, M. Buxton, et al. pp. 350–358. Boston: Schenkman.

Roszell, D. K., and Chaney, E. F. (1982). Autogenic training in a drug abuse program. *International Journal of the Addictions* 17(8): 1337–1349.

Rowe, D., and Grills, C. (1993). An alternative conceptual paradigm for drug counseling with African-American clients. *Journal of Psychoactive Drugs* 25(1):21–33.

Roy, C. (1973). Indian peyotists and alcohol. *American Journal Psychiatry* 130(3):329–330.

Roy, S., and Rizvi, S. H. M. (1987). Tribal hallucinogenic tradition: a case study of Manipur village. *Man in India* 87(2): 137–146.

Sainsbury, M. J. (1974). Acupuncture in heroin withdrawal. *Medical Journal of Australia* 2:102–105.

San Pedro, R. M., and Ponce, E. G. (1988). School programmes in drug rehabilitation and social reintegration in the Philippines. *Bulletin on Narcotics* 40(1):63–66.

Sandvig, A. (1991). Ungdom i graasonen—om samarbeid mellom frivillige organisasjoner skole og Tyrilikollektivet. [*Youth in the grey zone—concerning collaboration between volunteer organizations, schools and the tyrili collective.*] *Nota-Bene Rapport Nr.* 91:3.

Schmeck, H. (1977). Link between the human brain and opium poppy. *New Straits Times*, Kuala Lumpure, October 3. Reprinted from *The New York Times*.

Schuckit, M. A. (1989). Kava. *Drug Abuse and Alcoholism Newsletter* 18(2):1–3.

——— (1993). Acupuncture and the treatment of drug withdrawal syndromes. *Drug Abuse and Alcoholism Newsletter* 21:1–4.

Schultes, R. E. (1972). An overview of hallucinogens in the western hemisphere. In *Flesh of the Gods*, ed. P. T. Furst, pp. 3–54. New York: Praeger.

——— (1977). Mexico and Colombia: two major centres of aboriginal use of hallucinogens. *Journal of Psychedelic Drugs* 9(2): 173–176.

——— (1984). Fifteen years of study of psychoactive snuffs of South America: 1967–1982—a review. *Journal of Ethnopharmacology* 11:17–32.

Schuster, R. (1975). Meditation: philosophy and practice in a drug rehabilitation setting. *Forum* 5(2):163–170.

Severson, L., et al. (1977). Heroin detoxification and electrical stimulation. *International Journal of the Addiction* 12(7):911–922.

Shaffi, M., Lavely, R., and Jaffe, R. (1975). Meditation and the prevention of alcohol abuse. *American Journal of Psychiatry* 132:942–945.

Shanmugasundaram, E. R. B., and Shanmugasundaram, K. R. (1986). An Indian herbal formula (SKY) for controlling voluntary ethanol intake in rats with chronic alcoholism. *Journal of Ethnopharmacology* 17:171–182.

Sharma, K., and Shukla, V. (1988). Rehabilitation of drug-addicted persons: the experience of the Nav-Chetna Center in India. *Bulletin on Narcotics* 40(1):43–49.

Shrestha, N. M. (1992). Alcohol and drug abuse in Nepal. *British Journal of Addiction* 87:1241–1248.

Sidel, V., and Sidel, R. (1973). *Serve the People: Observations on Medicine in the People's Republic of China*. New York: J. Macy Foundation.

―――― (1974). The delivery of medical care in China. *Scientific American* 230(4):19–27.

Singer, M. (1982). Christian Science healing and alcoholism: an anthropological perspective. *Journal of Operational Psychiatry* 13(1):2–12.

Singer, M., and Borrero, M. G. (1984). Indigenous treatment for alcoholism: the case of Puerto Rican Spiritism. *Medical Anthropology* 8(4):248–273.

Skeat, W. W. (1900). *Malay Magic*. London: Macmillan.

Smith, D. E. (1994). AA recovery and spirituality: an addiction medicine perspective. *Journal of Substance Abuse Treatment* 11(2):111–112.

Smith, D. E., Buxton, M. E., Bilal, R., and Seymour, R. B. (1993). Cultural points of resistance to the 12-step recovery process. *Journal of Psychoactive Drugs* 25(1):97–108.

Smith, M. O. (1988a). Acupuncture treatment for crack: clinical survey of 1,500 patients treated. *American Journal of Acupuncture* 16(3):241–247.

—— (1988b). The Lincoln Hospital Acupuncture Drug Abuse Program—Testimony presented to Andrew Stein, President of the New York City Council, June 29.
Smith, M. O., and Khan, I. (1988). An acupuncture programme for the treatment of drug-addicted persons. *Bulletin on Narcotics* 40(1):35–41.
Snyder, S. H., Pert, C. B., and Pasternak, D. W. (1974). The opiate receptor. *Annals of Internal Medicine* 81:534–540.
Sorhaug, H. C. (1984a). Youth, Youth Culture, and Work with Youth. Oslo: Institutes of Work Research.
—— (1984b). *Ungdom, Ungdomskultur og Ungdomsarbeid*. [*Youth, Youth Culture and Youth Work.*] Oslo: Arbeidsforsknings-instituttene.
—— (1988). Identitet: Grenser, autonomi og avhengighet—Stoffmisbrak som eksempel. [Identity: frontiers, autonomy and dependency—addiction as an example.] *Alkoholpolitik—Tidskrift for nordisk alkoholforskning*. 5:31–39.
Spencer, C. P., Heggenhougen, H. K., and Navaratnam, V. (1980). Traditional therapies and the treatment of drug dependence in Southeast Asia. *American Journal of Chinese Medicine* 8(3):230–238.
Stensrud, A. (1985). *Revansj—Ei Bok om Tyrili Kollektivet*. [*Revenge—A Book about the Tyrili Collective.*] Brumundal, Norway: Fagbokforlaget.
Stensrud, M. K., and Lushbough, R. S. (1988). The implementation of an occupational therapy program in an alcohol and drug dependency treatment center. Special issue: Treatment and Substance Abuse: Psychosocial Occupational Therapy Approaches. *Occupational Therapy in Mental Health* 8(2):1–15.
Suwaki, H. (1979). "Naikan" and "Danshukai" for the treatment of Japanese alcoholic patients. *British Journal of the Addictions* 74:15–19.

——— (1980). Japan: culturally based treatment of alcoholism. In *Drug Problems in Sociocultural Context—A Basis for Policies and Programme Planning*, ed. G. Edwards and A. Arif, Public Health Papers No. 73, pp. 139–143. Geneva: WHO.

Suwanwela, C., and Poshyachinda, V. (1983). Thailand: rendering opium redundant. In *Drug Use and Misuse—Cultural Perspectives (Based on a Collaborative Study by the World Health Organization)*, ed. G. Edwards, A. Arif, and J. Jaffe, pp. 215–220. London: Croom Helm.

——— (1986). Drug abuse in Asia. *Bulletin on Narcotics* 38(1, 2): 41–53.

Szasz, T. (1977). The ethics of addiction. In *The Theology of Medicine*, ed. T. Szasz, pp. 29–48. New York: Harper & Row.

Thelander, A. (1979). *Hassela Kollektivet—En Rapport om Vardinnehall och Vardideologi pa ett Hem for Unga Narkomaner.* [*The Hassela Collective—A Report about Value Content and Value Ideology in a Home for Young Narcotic Addicts.*] Stokholm: Prisma.

Tiwari, V. J., Padhye, M. D., and Deshmukh, V. K. (1990). Plant hallucinogens and shaman. *Eastern Anthropologist* 43(4): 371–375.

Touchette, N. (1993). Ibogaine neurotoxicity raises new questions in addiction research. *Journal of NIH Research* 5: 50–55.

Trotter, R. T. (1979). Evidence of an ethnomedical form of aversion therapy on the United States-Mexico border. *Journal of Ethnopharmacology* 1:279–284.

Tyrili-Kollektivet (1989). *For Harde Livet!* [*It is a Matter of Life or Death.*] Aarsmellding (Annual Report). Tyrili, Norway: Tyrili-Kollektivet.

Vaglum, P. (1979). *Unge Stoffmisbrukere i et "Terapeutisk Samfunn"—Forlop under og efter Behandling. En Klinisk Psykiatrisk undersokelse.* [*Young Drug Abusers in a "Therapeutic Com-*

munity." Results during and after Therapy. A Clinical Psychiatric Investigation.] Oslo: Universitetsforlaget.
—— (1981). Miljoterapi av unge stoffmisbrukere i Norge. [Environmental therapy for young drug abusers in Norway.] *Tidskrift for den Norske Laegeforening* 14(101):852–855.
Valla, J.-P., and Prince, R. H. (1989). Religious experiences as self-healing mechanisms. In *Altered States of Consciousness and Mental Health—A Cross-Cultural Perspective*, ed. C. A. Ward, Cross-Cultural Research and Methodology Series, vol. 12, pp. 149–166. Newbury Park, CA: Sage.
Waal, H., Andresen, A. S., and Kaada, A. K. (1981). *Kollektiver—Hverdag og virkninger. [Collectives—Daily Process and Effect.]* Oslo: Universtitetsforlaget.
Wallace, R. K. (1970). Physiological effects of transcendental meditation. *Science* 167:1751–1754.
Wallace, R. K., and Benson, H. (1972). The physiology of meditation. *Scientific American* 226:84–90.
Ward, C. A. (1989a). The cross-cultural study of altered states of consciousness and mental health. In *Altered States of Consciousness and Mental Health—A Cross-Cultural Perspective*, ed. C. A. Ward, Cross-Cultural Research and Methodology Series, vol. 12, pp. 15–35. Newbury Park, CA: Sage.
——, ed. (1989b). *Altered States of Consciousness and Mental Health—A Cross-Cultural Perspective*, Cross-Cultural Research and Methodology Series, vol. 12. Newbury Park, CA: Sage.
Washburn, A. M., Fullilove, R. E., Fullilove, M. T., et al. (1993). Acupuncture heroin detoxification: a single-blind clinical trial. *Journal of Substance Abuse Treatment* 10:345–351.
Weibel-Orlando, J. C. (1984). Indian alcoholism treatment programs as flawed rites of passage. *Medical Anthropology Quarterly* 15(3):62–67.
Wen, H. L. (1980). Clinical experience and mechanism of acupuncture and electrical stimulation (AES) in the treatment

of drug abuse. *American Journal of Chinese Medicine* 8(4): 349–353.

Wen, H. L., and Cheung, S. Y. C. (1973). Treatment of drug addiction by acupuncture and electrical stimulation. *Asian Journal of Medicine* 9:138–141.

Westermeyer, J. (1971). Use of alcohol and opium among the Meo of Laos. *American Journal of Psychiatry* 124:1019–1023.

—— (1973). Folk treatment for opium addiction in Laos. *British Journal of Addiction* 68:345–349.

—— (1974). Opium smoking in Laos: a survey of 40 addicts. *American Journal of Psychiatry* 131:165–170.

—— (1977a). Narcotic addiction in two Asian cultures: a comparison and analysis. *Drug and Alcohol Dependence* 2:273–285.

—— (1977b). Opium and heroin addicts in Laos. *Journal of Nervous and Mental Disease* 164(5):346–354.

—— (1979). Medical and non medical treatment of narcotic addicts: a comparative study from Asia. *Journal of Nervous and Mental Disease* 167(4):205–211.

—— (1980). Treatment for narcotic addiction in a Buddhist monastery. *Journal of Drug Issues* 10:221–228.

—— (1989). Nontreatment factors affecting treatment outcome in substance abuse. *American Journal of Drug and Alcohol Abuse* 15(1):13–29.

Westermeyer, J., and Bourne, P. (1978). Treatment outcome and the role of the community in narcotic addiction. *Journal of Nervous and Mental Disease* 166:51–58.

Westermeyer, J., and Walzer, V. (1975). Drug usage: an alternative to religion? *Diseases of the Nervous System* 36(9): 492–495.

Whitehead, P. C. (1978). Acupuncture in the treatment of addiction: a review and analysis. *International Journal of the Addictions* 13(1):1–16.

WHO (1975). Training and utilization of traditional healers and their collaboration with heatlh care delivery systems, Executive Board, 57th Sessions, Provisional Agenda, Item 17, EB57/21 Add. 2, November 2.
—— (1976). Twenty-ninth World Health Assembly—1. *WHO Chronicle* 30:259–263.
—— (1977). Traditional medicine—views from South East Asia region. *WHO Chronicle* 31:47–52.
WHO/Unicef (1978). *Primary Health Care, Report of the International Conference on PHC.* Alma ATA, USSR. Geneva: WHO.
Winkler, A. (1974). Requirements for extinction of relapse facilitating variables and for rehabilitation in a narcotic antagonist treatment program. In *Narcotic Antagonists: Advances in Biochemical Pharmacology*, vol. 8, ed. M. C. Braude, et al., pp. 399–414. New York: Raven.
Wilson, P. (1987). The understanding of drug use, abuse and dependence, and its treatment by homeopathy and other therapies. Unpublished manuscript.
Wilson, W. P. (1972). Mental health benefits of religious salvation. *Diseases of the Nervous System* 33:382–386.
Wolff, R. J. (1965). Modern medicine and traditional culture: confrontation on the Malay peninsula. *Human Organization* 24:339.
Worner, T. M., Zeller, B., Schwarz, H., et al. (1992). Acupuncture fails to improve treatment outcome in alcoholics. *Drug and Alcohol Dependence* 30:169–173.
Yablonsky, L. (1989). *The Therapeutic Community: A Successful Approach for Treating Substance Abusers.* New York: Gardner.
Yang, M. M. P., and Kwok, J. S. L. (1986). Evaluation on the treatment of morphine addiction by acupuncture, Chinese herbs and opioid peptides. *American Journal of Chinese Medicine* 14(1, 2):46–50.
Yang, M. M. P., Yuen, R. C. F., and Kwok, J. S. L. (1985). Effect of

certain Chinese herbs on drug addiction. In *Advances in Chinese Medicinal Materials Research*, ed. H. M. Chang, H. W. Yeung, W. W. Tso, and A. Koo, pp. 147–158. Singapore: World Scientific Press.

Zinberg, N. E., Jacobsen, R. C., and Harding, W. M. (1975). Social sanctions and rituals as a basis for drug abuse prevention. *American Journal of Drug and Alcohol Abuse* 2(2): 165–182.

Zucker, D. K., Austin, F., Fair, A., and Branchey, L. (1987). Associations between patient religiosity and alcohol attitudes and knowledge in an alcohol treatment program. *International Journal of the Addictions* 22(1):47–53.

Zweben, J. E., ed. (1993). Culturally relevant substance abuse treatment. *Journal of Psychoactive Drugs* 25(1):1–108.

Supplemental Reading

Abrams, A. I., and Siegel, L. M. (1978). The transcendental meditation program and rehabilitation at Folsom State Prison: a cross-validation study. *Criminal Justice Behavior* 5:3–20.

Abu el Azayem, G. M. (1987). A psycho-socio-religious approach to contain substance abuse in Egypt. In *Congress Proceedings*, pp. 409–415. Lahore, Pakistan: World Islamic Association for Mental Health.

Achterberg, J. (1988). The wounded healer: transformational journeys in modern medicine. *Shaman's Drum*, Winter, pp. 19–24.

Adelman, E., and Castricone, L. (1986). An expressive arts model for substance abuse group training and treatment. *The Arts in Psychotherapy* 13:53–59.

Albert-Puleo, N. (1980). Modern psychoanalytic art therapy and its application to drug abuse. *The Arts in Psychotherapy* 7(1):43–52.

Allen, P. B. (1985). Integrating art therapy into an alcoholism treatment program. *American Journal of Art Therapy* 24:10–12.

Aron, A., and Aron, E. N. (1980). The transcendental meditation programme's effect on addictive behaviour. *Addictive Behaviours* 5:3–12.

Aron, E. N., and Aron, A. (1983). The patterns of reduction of drug and alcohol use among transcendental mediation participants. *Bulletin of the Society of Psychologists in Addictive Behaviors* 2:28–33.

Baasher, T. (1967). Traditional psychotherapeutic practices in the Sudan. *Transcultural Psychiatric Research Review* 4:158–160.

Baasher, T., and Abu el Azayem, G. M. (1980). Egypt (2): the role of the mosque in treatment in drug problems in the sociocultural context: a basis for policies and program planning. In *Public Health Paper No. 73*, ed. G. Edwards, pp. 131–134. Geneva: World Health Organization.

Bacon, S. (1985). *Outward Bound and Alcoholism and Drug Addiction.* Glenwood Springs, CO: Unpublished manuscript.

Benson, H., and Wallace, R. K. (1977). Decreased drug abuse with transcendental meditation: a study of 1862 subjects. In *Scientific Research on the Transcendental Meditation Program. Collected Papers*, vol. 1, ed. D. W. Orme-Johnson and J. T. Farrow. Weggis: Maharishi European Research University Press.

Blum, K., and Trachtenberg, M. (1986). Neurochemistry and alcohol craving. *California Society for the Treatment of Alcoholism and Other Drug Dependencies News* 13(2):1–7.

Bradshaw, J. (1988). *Healing the Shame That Binds You.* Deerfield Beach, FL: Health Communications.

Browne, G. E., et al. (1977). Improved mental and physical health and decreased use of prescribed and non-prescribed drugs through the transcendental meditation programme. In *Scientific Research on the Transcendental Meditation Program, Collected Papers*, vol. 3, ed. D. W. Orme-Johnson and J. T. Farrow. Weggis, Switzerland: Maharishi European Research University Press.

Bullock, M. L., Umen, A. J., Culliton, P. D., and Olander, R. T.

(1987). Acupuncture treatment of alcoholic recidivism: a pilot study. *Alcoholism (NY)* 11:292–295.

Cheng, R. S. S., Pomeranz, B., and Yu, G. (1980). Electroacupuncture treatment of morphine-dependent mice reduces signs of withdrawal without showing cross-tolerance. *European Journal of Pharmacology* 68:477.

Chiappe, M., Campos Fuentes, J., and Dragunsky, L. (1972). Psiquiatria folklorica peruana: el tratamiento del alcoholismo. *Acta Psichiatrica Psicologica de America Latina* 18: 385–394.

Craycroft, L., and Margoliash, L. (1972). WhiteBird Clinic: one way to prevent drug abuse. *Edcentric* 4(1):29–31.

Dillbeck, M. C., et al. (1987). Consciousness as a field: the transcendental meditation and TM-Sidhi programme and changes in social indicators. *Journal of Mind and Behavior* 8:67–103.

Dodes, L. M. (1990). Addiction, helplessness, and narcissistic rage. *Psychoanalytic Quarterly* 59:398–419.

Dougherty, P. M., and Dafny, N. (1989). Trans-cranial electrical stimulation attenuates the severity of naloxone-precipitated morphine withdrawal in rats. *Life Sciences* 44(2):2051–2056.

Efron, D. H., Holmstedt, B., and Kline, N. S., eds. (1967). *Ethnopharmacologic Search for Psychoactive Drugs*. Public Health Service Publication, No. 1645. Washington, DC: U.S. Government Printing Office. (Reprinted, New York: Raven Press, 1979.)

Ellison, F., Ellison, W., Daulouede, J. P., et al. (1987). Opiate withdrawal and electrostimulation. Double Blind experiments. *L'Encephale* 13:225–229.

Foulke, W. E., and Keller, T. W. (1976). The art experience in addict rehabilitation. *American Journal of Art Therapy* 15 (3):75–80.

Fraioli, F., Moreffl, C., Poolucci, D., et al. (1980). Physical exer-

cise stimulates marked concomitant release of beta-endorphin and adrenocorticotropic hormone (AcIti) in peripheral blood in man. *Experiential* 36:987–989.
Free, V., and Sanders, P. (1979). The use of ascorbic acid and mineral supplements in the detoxification of narcotic addicts. *Journal of Psychedelic Drugs* 11(3):217–222.
Gallardo de Parejo, J. (1986). New morning for Colombian youth. In *Bridging Services: Proceedings of the Ninth World Conference of Therapeutic Communities*. San Francisco: Abacus.
Gariti, P., Auriacombe, M., Inemikoski, R., et al. (1992). A randomized double-blind study of neuroelectric therapy in opiate and cocaine detoxification. *Journal of Substance Abuse* 4(3):299–308.
Gibson, M. (1980). The Outward Bound experience: a new and unique humanistic approach for the treatment of alcoholism. In *Outward Bound in Alcohol Treatment and Mental Health: A Compilation of Literature*, ed. T. Stich. Greenwich, CT: Outward Bound.
Gordon, A. (1981). The cultural context of drinking and indigenous therapy for alcohol problems in three migrant Hispanic cultures. *Journal of Studies on Alcohol* 9(suppl): 217–240.
Gossop, M., Strang, J., and Connell, P. (1984). Electrostimulation and methadone withdrawal. *British Journal of Psychiatry* 144:203–208.
Gouterel, R., Gollnhofer, O., and Sillans, R. (1993). Pharmacodynamics and therapeutic applications of iboga and ibogaine. *Psychedelic Monograph Essays* 6:71.
Grinenko, A., Krupitskiy, E. M., Lebedev, V. P., et al. (1988). Metabolism of biogenic amines during the treatment of alcohol withdrawal syndrome by transcranial electric treatment. *Biogenic Amines* 5(6):427–436.

Gunther, E. (1949). The Shaker religion of the northwest. In *Indians of the Urban Northwest*, ed. M. W. Smith, pp. 37–76. New York: Columbia University Press.

Hall, R., (1986). Alcohol treatment in American Indian populations: an indigenous treatment modality compared with traditional approaches. *Annals of the New York Academy of Sciences* 472:168–178.

Han, J., and Shai, L. S. (1990). Differential release of enkephalin and dynorphin by low and high frequency electroacupuncture. *Acupuncture* 1:1–9.

Han, J., Tang, J., Huang, B., et al. (1979). Acupuncture tolerance in rats: anti-opiate substrate implicated. *Chinese Medical Journal* 9(9):625–627.

Harner, M. (1980a). *The Way of the Shaman*. New York: Bantam.

—— (1980b). *The Way of the Shaman/A Guide to Power and Healing*. New York: Harper & Row.

Hay, D. (1980). *The phenomology of spontaneous religious experience*. Paper presented at Shamans and Endorphins Conference, Montreal.

Hiegel, J. P. (1988). *Opium detoxification of Lao hill tribe refugees in the Phanat Nikhom Camp*. Paper presented at the 11th World Conference of Therapeutic Communities, Bangkok, Thailand, February.

Ho, W. K. K., Wen, H. L., Lam, S., and Ma, L. (1978). The influence of electroacupuncture on naloxone-induced morphine withdrawal in mice: evaluation of brain opiate-like activity. *European Journal of Pharmacology* 49(2):197–199.

James, M. R. (1988). Music therapy and alcoholism: II. Treatment services. *Music Therapy Perspectives* 5:65–68.

James, M. R., and Townsley, R. K. (1989). Activity therapy services and chemical dependency rehabilitation. *Journal of Alcohol and Drug Education* 34:48–53.

Jilek, W. (1976). Brain washing as a therapeutic technique in contemporary Canadian Indian spirit dancing. In *Anthropology and Mental Health*, ed. J. Westermeyer, pp. 201–213. The Hague: Mouton.

—— (1981). Anomic depression, alcoholism and a culture-congenial Indian response. *Journal of Studies on Alcohol* 9(suppl):159–170.

—— (1982). *Indian Healing: Shamanic Ceremonialism in the Pacific Northwest Today*. Surrey, British Columbia: Hancock House.

Jilek-Aall, L. (1981). Acculturation, alcoholism and Indian-style alcoholics anonymous. *Journal of Studies on Alcohol* 9(suppl):143–158.

Karrell, R. (1990). Acupuncture in an adolescent treatment setting. *Addiction and Recovery* 10:24–27.

Katz, D. (1976). Decreased drug use and the prevention of drug use through the transcendental meditation programme. In *Collected Papers*, vol. 1, pp. 536–543. Rheinweiler: MERU Press.

Kaufman, G. H. (1981). Art therapy with the addicted. *Journal of Psychoactive Drugs* 13(4):353–360.

Khalsa, D. R., and Singh, S. (1977). Ascent from addiction. *New Directions* 26:17–18.

Kosterlitz, H. W., and Hughes, J. (1975). Some thoughts on the significance of enkephalin, the endogenous ligand. *Life Sciences* 17:91–96.

Kraus, A. R. (1956). *Short-term relaxation therapy with groups of non-psychotic alcoholics*. Paper presented at the Fourth Inter-American Congress of Psychology, University of Puerto Rico.

Krupitsky, E. M., Burakov, A. M., Karandashova, G. F., et al. (1991). The administration of transcranial electric treatment for affective disturbances therapy in alcoholic patients. *Drug and Alcohol Dependence* 27:1–6.

LaBarre, W. (1938). *The Peyote Cult.* Publications in Anthropology No. 19. New Haven: Yale University.
—— (1964). The narcotic complex of the New World. *Diogenes* 48:125–138.
—— (1970). Review of R. G. Wasson, Soma. *American Anthropologist* 72:368–373.
Lake, J. R., Brubaker, D., Murray, J. B., et al. (1988). Transcranial electrostimulation (TCET) reduces pain sensitivity and opiate abstinence signs. *Physics in Medicine and Biology* 33(suppl 1):398.
Lipton, D. S., Brewington, V., and Smith, M. (1990). Acupuncture and crack addicts: a single-blind placebo test of efficacy. (NIDA Grant No. 1 RO1 DA05632-01; available from Narcotic and Drug Research, Inc., 11 Beach Street, New York, NY 10010.)
Lorini, G., Fazio, L., Cocchi, R., et al. (1979). Acupuncture as a part of a program of detoxification and weaning from opiates: 25 cases. *Minerva Medica* 70(56):3831–3836.
Low, S. A. (1974). Acupuncture and heroin withdrawal. *Medical Journal of Australia* 2:341.
Luzzatto, P. (1989). Drinking problems and short-term art therapy: working with images of withdrawal and clinging. In *Pictures at an Exhibition*, ed. A. Gilroy and T. Dalley, pp. 207–219. London: Tavistock/Routledge.
Mala, T. (1985). Alaska native grass roots movement: problem solving utilizing indigenous values. *Arctic Medical Research* 40:84–91.
Marcus, J. B. (1974). Transcendental meditation: a new method of reducing drug abuse. *Drug Forum* 3:113–136.
Marlatt, G. A., and Marques, J. K. (1977). Meditation, self control and alcohol use. In *Behavioral Self-Management: Strategies, Techniques and Outcomes*, ed. R. B. Stuart. New York: Brunner/Mazel.

Marlatt, G. A., and Nathan, P. E., eds. (1978). *Behavioral Approaches to Alcoholism*. New Brunswick, NJ: Rutgers Center of Alcohol Studies, pp. 222.

Mercer, G. W., and Smart, R. G. (1974). The epidemiology of psychoactive and hallucinogenic drug use. In *Research Advances in Alcohol and Drug Problems*, vol. 1, pp. 303–354. New York: Wiley.

Monahan, R. J. (1977). Secondary prevention of drug dependence through the transcendental meditation programme in metropolitan Philadelphia. *International Journal of the Addictions* 12:729–754.

Moore, R. W. (1983). Art therapy with substance abusers: a review of the literature. *The Arts in Psychotherapy* 10:251–260.

Murphy, M. (1983). Music therapy: a self-help group experience for substance abuse patients. *Music Therapy* 3:52–62.

National Council Against Health Fraud (1991). Acupuncture: the position paper of the National Council Against Health Fraud. *American Journal of Acupuncture* 19:273–279.

Ng, L. K. Y. (1975). Modification of morphine-withdrawal syndrome in rats following transauricular electrostimulation: an experimental paradigm for auricular electroacupuncture. *Biological Psychiatry* 10(5):575–580.

Nidich, S. I. (1980). *The science of creative intelligence and the transcendental meditation programme: reduction of drug and alcohol consumption*. Paper presented at the New England Educational Research Organization Conference, Lenox, Massachusetts.

Orme, M. E. J., and Snider, J. G. (1964). Autogenic training in the treatment of alcoholism. *Quarterly Journal of Studies in Alcohol* 25:547–550.

Orme-Johnson, D. W. (1987). Medical care utilization and the transcendental meditation programme. *Psychosomatic Medicine* 49:493–507.

Orme-Johnson, D. W., and Farrow, J. T., eds. (1977). *Scientific Research on the Transcendental Meditation Program: Collected Papers*, vols. 1–5. Weggis, Switzerland: Maharishi European Research University Press.

Parker, J. C., Gilbert, G. S., and Thoreson, R. W. (1978). Reduction of automatic arousal in alcoholics: a comparison of relaxation and meditation techniques. *Journal of Consulting and Clinical Psychology* 46:879–886.

Patterson, G., and Patterson, M. (1987). *The Power Factor*. Irving, TX: Word Publishing.

—— (1993). *The Paradise Factor*. Irving, TX: Word Publishing.

Patterson, M. A. (1978). The significance of current frequency in neuroelectric therapy (NET) for drug and alcohol addictions. In *Electrotherapeutic Sleep and Electroanaesthesia*, ed. F. M. Wageneder and R. H. Germann, pp. 285–296. Graz: RM Verlag.

—— (1986). *Hooked? NET: The New Approach to Drug Cure*. London, Boston: Faber & Faber.

Patterson, M., Firth, J., and Gardiner, R. (1984). Treatment of drug, alcohol and nicotine addiction by neuroelectricity therapy: analysis of results over 7 years. *Journal of Bioelectricity* 3:193–221.

Peele, S. (1975). *Love and Addiction*. New York: Signet.

Peng, C. H., Yang, M. M., Kok, S. H., and Woo, Y. K. (1978). Endorphin release: a possible mechanism of acupuncture analgesia. *Comparative Medicine East/West* 6(1): 57–60.

Pert, C. B. (1986). The window of the receptors: neuropeptides, the emotions, and body mind. *Advances* 3:8–16.

Pert, C. B., Ruff, M. R., Weba, R. J., and Herkenharn, M. (1985). Neuropeptides and their receptors: a psychosomatic network. *Journal of Immunology* 135:820–826.

Peters, L. (1981). *Ecstasy and Healing in Negal*. Malibu: Undena.

Pomeranz, B., and Chiu, D. (1976). Naloxone blockade of acupuncture analgesia: endorphin implicated. *Life Sciences* 19:1757–1762.

Reynolds, K. (1977). Naikan therapy—an experimental view. *International Journal of Social Psychiatry* 23:252–264.

Rice, B. (1979). Will herb tea replace methadone? *Psychology Today*, March.

Rohsenow, D. J., Smith, R. E., and Johnson, S. (1985). Stress management training as a prevention program for heavy social drinkers: cognitions, affect drinking and individual differences. *Addiction Behavior* 10:45–54.

Ruiz, P., and Langrod, J. (1984). Spiritual healing and family therapy. *Common Approaches to the Treatment of Alcoholism Family Therapy* 11(2):155–162.

Sacks, L. (1975). Drug addiction, alcoholism, smoking, obesity treated by auricular staple-puncture. *American Journal of Acupuncture* 3:147–150.

Schneider, J. A., and McArthur, M. (1956). Potentiation action of ibogaine (Bogadin TM) on morphine analgesia. *Experientia* 8:323.

Schultes, R. E., and Hofmann, A. (1979). *Plants of the Gods*. New York: McGraw-Hill.

Scott, S. (1983). A holistic approach to medical treatment for cocaine dependent clients. *Cocaine Connection* 1:2–3.

Shafii, M., Lavely, R. A., and Jaffe, R. D. (1974). Meditation and marijuana. *American Journal of Psychiatry* 131:60–63.

—— (1975). Meditation and the prevention of alcohol abuse. *American Journal of Psychiatry* 132:242–245.

Sharps, H. (1977). Acupuncture and the treatment of drug withdrawal symptoms. *PharmChem Newsletter* 6(7):1–6.

Sjolund, B., and Eriksson, M. (1976). Electroacupuncture and endogenous morphines. *Lancet* 2:1085.

Smith, D. E., and Gay, G. R. (1972). *It's So Good Don't Even Try It Once*. Englewood Cliffs, NJ: Prentice-Hall.

Smith, M. (1978). *Natural healing and drug detoxification*. Paper presented at the National Drug Abuse Conference, Seattle.

—— (1979). Acupuncture and natural healing in drug detoxification. *American Journal of Acupuncture* 2(7):97–106.

Smith, M. O., Squires, R., Aponte, J., et al. (1982). Acupuncture treatment of drug addiction and alcohol abuse. *American Journal of Acupuncture* 10:161–163.

Spoth, R. (1980). Using a differential stress reduction model with substance abuses: matching treatment presentation with locus of control. *Behavior Analysis and Modification* 4:188–200.

Stark, M. J. (1989). A psychoeducational approach to methadone maintenance treatment. *Journal of Substance Abuse Treatment* 6(3):169–181.

Stefaniszyn, B. (1964). *Social and Ritual Life of the Ambo of Northern Rhodesia*. London: Oxford University Press.

Stich, T., ed. (1984). *Outward Bound in Alcohol Treatment and Mental Health: A Compilation of Literature*. Greenwich, CT: Outward Bound.

Strickler, D. P., Tomaszewski, R., Maxwell, W. A., and Suib, M. B. (1979). The effects of relaxation instructions on drinking behavior in the presence of stress. *Behavior Research and Therapy* 17:45–51.

Tarbox, A. R. (1983). Alcoholism, biofeedback and internal scanning. *Journal of Studies in Alcohol* 44(2):246–261.

Tennant, F. (1976). Outpatient heroin detoxification with acupuncture and staplepuncture. *Western Journal of Medicine* 125:191–194.

TerRiet, G., Kleijnen, J., and Knipschild, P. (1990). A meta-analysis of studies into the effect of acupuncture on addiction. *British Journal of General Practice* 40:379–382.

Trotter, R. T., and Chavira, I. A. (1978). Discovering new models for alcohol counseling in minority group. In *Modern Medicine and Medical Anthropology in the United States-Mexico Border Population*, ed. B. Velimirovic, pp. 164–171. Washington, DC: Pan American Health Organization.

Turner, V. (1974). *Dramas, Fields, and Metaphors. Symbolic Action in Human Society.* Ithaca, NY: Cornell University Press.

Wadden, T. A., and Penrod, J. H. (1981). Hypnosis in the treatment of alcoholism: a review and appraisal. *American Journal of Clinical Hypnosis* 24:41–47.

Wallace, A. F. C. (1958). Dreams and the wishes of the soul: a type of psychoanalytic theory among the seventeenth century Iroquois. *American Anthropologist* 60:234–248.

—— (1966). *Religion: An Anthropological View*. New York: Random House.

Wallace, R. K. (1977). The physiological effects of transcendental meditation: a proposed fourth major state of consciousness. In *Scientific Research on the Transcendental Meditation Program Collected Papers*, vol. 1, ed. D. W. Orme-Johnson and J. T. Farrow. Weggis, Switzerland: Maharishi European Research University Press.

Wallace, R. K., and Benson, H. (1972). Decreased drug abuse with transcendental meditation: a study of 1,862 subjects. In *Drug Abuse: Proceedings of the International Conference*, ed. J. D. Zarafonetis, pp. 369–376. Philadelphia: Lea and Febiger.

Weil, A., and Rosen, W. (1993). *From Chocolate to Morphine: Everything You Need to Know about Mind-Altering Drugs.* Boston: Houghton Mifflin.

Wen, H. L. (1977). Fast detoxification of drug abuse by acupuncture and electrical stimulation (A. E. S.) in combination with naloxone. *Modern Medicine Asia* 13:13–17.

Wen, H. L., and Cheung, S. Y. C. (1973). How acupuncture can help addicts. *Drugs and Society* 2:8–18.

Wen, H. L., Ng, Y. H., Ho, W. K. K., et al. (1978). Acupuncture in narcotic withdrawal: a preliminary report on biochemical changes in the blood and urine of heroin addicts. *Bulletin on Narcotics* 30(2):31–39.

Wen, H. L., and Teo, S. W. (1975). Experience in the treatment of drug addiction by electroacupuncture. *Modern Medicine in Asia* 11:23–24.

Whitfield, C. (1984). Stress management and spirituality during recovery: a transpersonal approach. *Alcoholism Treatment Quarterly* 1:3–54.

Winquist, W. T. (1977). The transcendental meditation program and drug abuse: a retrospective study. In *Scientific Research on the Transcendental Meditation Program. Collected Papers*, vol. 1, ed. D. W. Orme-Johnson, and J. T. Farrow. Weggis, Switzerland: Maharishi European Research University Press.

Wong, M. R., Brochin, N. E., and Gendron, K. L. (1981). Effects of meditation on anxiety and chemical dependency. *Journal of Drug Education* 11:91–105.

Zuroff, D. C., and Schwarz, J. C. (1978). Effects of transcendental meditation and muscle relaxation on trait anxiety, maladjustment, locus of control, and drug use. *Journal of Consulting and Clinical Psychology* 46:264–271.

Credits

The author gratefully acknowledges permission to reprint material from the following:

"Understanding the High Mind" by K. Blum and J. E. Tilton, in *Folk Medicine and Herbal Healing*, ed. G. G. Meyer, K. Blum, and J. G. Cull, pp. 261–274. Copyright © 1981 by Charles C Thomas.

"Culture and Community in Therapeutic Community: Implications for the Treatment of Recovering Substance Misusers" by S. D. Christie and S. T. DeBerry, in *International Journal of the Addictions* 29(6):803–817. Copyright © 1994 by Marcel Dekker, Inc.

"Hallucinogenic Plants and Their Use in Traditional Societies—An Overview" by W. Davis, in *Cultural Survival Quarterly* 9(4):2–5. Copyright © 1985 by *Cultural Survival Quarterly*.

"Innovative Addiction Treatment: A Combination of Traditional Therapy and a Wilderness-Based Program" by M. K. Houston and A. Drum, in ICAA, *31st International Institute on the Prevention and Treatment of Alcoholism*. Proceedings, vol. 2, ed. E. Tongue and A. Tongue, pp. 89–103. Rome, Italy, 1985. Copyright © 1990 by the International Council on Alcohol and Addictions.

"Native Renaissance: The Survival and Revival of Indigenous Therapeutic Ceremonials among North American Indians" by W. G. Jilek, in *Transcultural Psychiatric Research* 15:117–147. Copyright © 1978 by *Transcultural Psychiatric Research*.

"Traditional Medicine Relevant to Psychiatry" by W. G. Jilek, in *Treatment of Mental Disorders*, ed. N. Sartorius, G. de Girolamo, G. Andrews, et al., pp. 341–390. Copyright © 1993 by World Health Organization.

"Creative Therapies in the Treatment of Addictions: The Art of Transforming Shame" by L. Johnson, in *The Arts in Psychotherapy* 17:299–308. Copyright © 1990 by Elsevier Science Ltd.

"Herbal Therapy in the Treatment of Drug Use" by E. Nebelkopf, in *International Journal of the Addictions* 22(8):695–717. Copyright © 1987 by Marcel Dekker, Inc.

"Herbs and Substance Abuse Treatment: A 10-Year Perspective" by E. Nebelkopf, in *Psychoactive Drugs* 20(3): 349–354. Copyright © 1988 by Haight-Ashbury Publications.

"A Review on the Buddhist Temple Drug Dependence Treatment in Thailand" by V. Poshyachinda. Paper presented at the meeting of WHO Substance Abuse Collaborating Centres, Geneva, September. Copyright © 1993 by V. Poshyachinda.

"Indigenous Treatment for Alcoholism: The Case of Puerto Rican Spiritism" by M. Singer and M. G. Borrero, in *Medical Anthropology* 8(4):248–273. Copyright © 1984 by *Medical Anthropology*.

"Cultural Points of Resistance to the 12-Step Recovery Process" by D. E. Smith, M. E. Buxton, R. Bilal, and R. B. Seymour, in *Journal of Psychoactive Drugs* 25(1):97–108. Copyright © 1993 by Haight-Ashbury Publications.

"Ibogaine Neurotoxicity Raises New Questions in Addiction Research" by N. Touchette, in *Journal of NIH Research* 5:50–55. Copyright © 1993 by *The Journal of NIH Research*.

Evidence of an Ethnomedical Form of Aversion Therapy on the United States-Mexico Border" by R. T. Trotter, in *Journal of Ethnopharmacology* 1:279–284. Copyright © 1979 by Elsevier Science Ireland Ltd.

"Effect of Certain Chinese Herbs on Drug Addiction" by M. M. P. Yang, R. C. F. Yuen, and J. S. L. Kwok, in *Advances in Chinese Medicinal Materials Research*, ed. H. M. Chang, H. W. Yeung, W. W. Tso, and A. Koo, pp. 147–158. Copyright © 1985 by World Scientific Publishing Co. Pte. Ltd.

"Social Sanctions and Rituals as a Basis for Drug Abuse Prevention" by N. E. Zinberg, R. C. Jacobsen, and W. M. Harding, in *American Journal of Drug and Alcohol* 2(2):165–182. Copyright © 1975 by Marcel Dekker, Inc.

Index

Abdul Rashid bin Abdul Razak, 24, 28
Abn el Azayem, G. M., 14
Acupuncture, 5, 12–13
　bibliography on, 95–101
　described, 81–86
Affect, bibliography on, 103–104
African Americans, spiritualism, 73, 75–76
Agar, M., 7
Albaugh, B. J., 52
Alcoholics Anonymous (AA), 60, 70, 72
Alcoholism treatment
　herbal, 42–43
　peyote rituals, 51–58
Alienation, as cause, 59
Altered states of consciousness therapy (ASCT)
　bibliography on, 106–110
　Native Americans, 56
Alternative therapies. *See also* Traditional medicine
　acupuncture, 81–86
　biofeedback, 67–68
　features of, 87–91

　implications of, for future programs, 91–92
　meditation, 69–72
　overview of, 5–6
　ritual, 77–80
　spiritualism, 72–77
　therapeutic communities, 59–66
Anderson, D., 11, 71
Anderson, P. O., 52
Andresen, A. S., 63
Arif, A., 87
Arokiasamy, C. M. V., 23
Art therapy
　bibliography on, 139–140
　described, 64–66

Baasher, T. A., 14
Baer, H. A., 10, 75, 76, 77
Behavior, bibliography on, 103–104
Benson, H., 10, 11, 69
Bergman, R. L., 52
Bibliotherapy
　bibliography on, 139–140
　described, 66

Bihari, B., 84
Biofeedback, 72
 bibliography on, 111–112
 described, 67–68
Blum, K., 11, 53, 56
Borrero, M. G., 73, 74, 75
Bourne, P. G., 10
Bowers, J. Z., 6
Bradshaw, J., 65
Bressler, M. J., 72
Brinkman, D. N., 68
Brown, J. K., 68
Brumbaugh, A. G., 83, 85
Buckley, P., 10, 71
Buddhism, Thailand, 35–39
Bullock, M. L., 83, 84
Burkill, I. H., 15, 18, 22
Buxton, M. E., 10, 67, 72

Cappendijk, S. L. T., 46
Carrubba, R. W., 6
Chaney, E. F., 68
Chen, J. Y. P., 9
Chen, P. C. Y., 17, 18
Cheung, S. Y. C., 5, 12, 81
Chinese medicine, Malaysia, 17–18
Christian Science, 76–77
Christie, S. D., 60, 61, 62
Clements, G., 10, 11, 67, 69
Colson, A. C., 18
Cowley, G., 45
Crawford, R. J. M., 72
Creative writing, described, 65–66

Daytop Village, 60
DeBerry, S. T., 60, 61, 62

Deecher, D. C., 46
Denney, M. R., 10, 68
DeRios, M. D., 78, 79
deSilva, P., 14
Drama therapy
 bibliography on, 139–140
 described, 65
Drug abuse
 causes of, 8
 extent of, 3
 historical perspective on, 6–9
 sociocultural context of, 3–4
Drum, A., 62
Dunn, F. L., 10, 16, 17
Dushman, R. D., 72
Dzoljif, M. R., 46

Edwards, G., 87
Emboden, W. A., 15, 78
Engelmajer, L. J., 63
Equinox Group, 82

Fernandez, J. W., 44
Follow-up studies
 Malaysia, 23–34
 Thailand, 38–39
Furst, P. T., 6, 78
Furuholmen, D., 63
Futterman, S., 53, 54

Galanter, M., 10, 71
Ganguli, H. C., 71
Gaylin, W., 60
Gelderloos, P., 11, 69, 70
Gimlette, J. D., 15, 18, 21, 22

Glick, S. D., 46
Gourd Dance, 48–49
Graves, R., 65
Greve, J., 63

Hallucinogens
  bibliography on, 106–110
  Peyote rituals, 51–58
Hamarneh, S., 6
Haniff, M., 15, 18, 22
Hare, H. A., 17
Harner, M. J., 6
Heggenhougen, H. K., 16, 18, 19, 24, 25, 26, 31, 35
Herbal treatments
  bibliography on, 123–128
  ibogaine, 44–46
  overview of, 41–44
  Thailand, 38
Hill, T. W., 11, 53
Houston, M. K., 62
Howard, J. H., 47

Ibogaine
  bibliography on, 125–128
  herbal treatments, 44–46

Jilek, W. G., 10, 12, 35, 47, 48, 49, 50, 51
Jilek-Aall, L., 35
Johnson, L., 64
Jung, C. G., 72

Kao, A. A., 12, 13, 82, 85
Khan, I., 9, 82, 83, 84, 85, 86
Klajner, F., 68
Kwok, J. S. L., 83

LaBarre, W., 6, 15, 22
Lamontagne, Y., 67
LaSalvia, T. A., 64
Latinos, spiritualism, 73–75
Lau, M. P., 12, 82
Lee, R. L. M., 23
Lex, B. W., 11, 12, 30
Lowinger, P., 7
Lu, L. Y. C., 12, 13, 82, 85
Lushbough, R. S., 64

Mahony, J., 66
Maisonneuve, I. M., 46
Mala, T. A., 14
Malaysia, 15–34
  bibliography on, 113–121
  Chinese medicine, 17–18
  follow-up studies in, 23–34
  overview, 15–16
  traditional medicine of, 18–23
Margolin, A., 82, 83
Martin, R. T., 6
Marx, J. L., 11
McBride, C. A., 17
McCoy, A., 7
McDonald, E., 66
McKay, D. A., 19
McLelland, A. T., 85
McPeake, J. D., 56, 57
Meditation
  bibliography on, 129–131
  described, 69–72
  rehabilitation and, 11
Menninger, K., 52
Meyer, R., 11, 30
Mohd. Taib Osman, 18, 19
Morinis, E. A., 10

Music therapy, bibliography on, 139–140

National Institute for Drug Abuse (NIDA), 84
Native American Church, peyote rituals, 51–58
Native Americans, 47–58
  overview, 47–51
  peyote rituals, 51–58
Navaratnam, V., 24, 25, 31
Nebelkopf, E., 41, 42, 43
Negrete, J. C., 6
Nelson, G. R., 10
Newmeyer, J. A., 82

Opiate use/abuse, historical perspective on, 6–9
Outward Bound
  bibliography on, 149–153
  described, 59, 62–63, 66

Pardeck, J. T., 66
Pascarosa, P., 53, 54
Patterson, M. A., 11, 12, 81, 82, 83, 85, 86
Peele, S., 61
Pelletier, K. R., 11
Petersen, R. C., 6
Peyote rituals, 51–58
Phoenix House, 60
Pigot, R., 57
Poetry, described, 65
Politics, drug abuse and, 4–5
Poshyachinda, V., 35, 38, 39
Prabhakaran, L. G., 23
Preeja, P., 36
Prince, R. H., 10, 11, 12, 57, 78

Psychodrama
  bibliography on, 139–140
  described, 72
Psychoeducation, 64
Psychology, bibliography on, 103–104
Public health perspective, drug abuse and, 4–5

Quinn, J. R., 9

Recidivism rates. *See* Follow-up studies
Relaxation therapy, bibliography on, 111–112
Religion
  bibliography on, 141–144
  Buddhism, Thailand, 35–39
  Malaysia, 19–20
  peyote rituals, 51–58
  rehabilitation and, 10–11
  spiritualism, described, 72–77
Revivalism, bibliography on, 141–144
Richards, L. G., 10
Ridley, H. N., 19
Riet, G. T., 13, 84
Ripinsky-Naxon, M., 10, 78
Ritual
  bibliography on, 141–144
  described, 77–80
Roman, Y. M., 55, 67
Roszell, D. K., 68
Roy, C., 52

Sainsbury, M. J., 12, 82
Sandvig, A., 63
Schmeck, H., 13

Schor, N., 11, 12
Schuckit, M. A., 85
Schultes, R. E., 6
Schuster, R., 10, 11
Severson, L., 13
Shaffi, M., 11
Shamans, bibliography on, 145–147
Shame, art therapy and, 64–65
Sharma, K., 14
Shukla, V., 14
Sidel, R., 9
Sidel, V., 9
Singer, M., 10, 73, 74, 75, 76
Skeat, W. W., 19
Smith, D. E., 10, 72, 78, 79
Smith, M. O., 9, 82, 83, 84, 85, 86
Snyder, S. H., 11
Southeast Asia, bibliography on, 113–121
Spiritualism
 bibliography on, 141–144
 described, 72–77
Stensrud, M. K., 64
Sun Dance, 49
Suwaki, H., 11, 14
Suwanwela, G., 35
Synanon, 60

Taricone, P. T., 23
Thailand, 35–39
 bibliography on, 113–121
 follow-up studies, 38–39
 treatments, 35–38
Therapeutic communities
 bibliography on, 149–153
 described, 59–66

Thomson, H. W., 15, 21, 22
Tilton, J. E., 11, 56
Tiwari, V. J., 78
Touchette, N., 46
Traditional medicine. *See also* Alternative therapies
 bibliography on, 155–160
 herbal treatments, 41–46
 Malaysia, 15–34. *See also* Malaysia
 Native American, 47–58. *See also* Native Americans
 overview of, 9–14
 Thailand, 35–39. *See also* Thailand
Transcendental meditation. *See* Meditation
Treatment, traditional medicine and, 9–14. *See also* Alternative therapies; Traditional medicine
Trotter, R. T., 41, 44

U Khant, 13

Vaglum, P., 63
Valla, J. P., 10, 11, 12, 57

Waal, H., 63
Wallace, R. K., 11, 69
Waller, D., 66
Walzer, V., 10
Washburn, A. M., 85
Wen, H. L., 5, 12, 81, 83
Westermeyer, J., 10
Whitehead, C., 82
Whitehead, P. C., 13, 83, 84
Winkler, A., 30

Winter Spirit Dance, 50
Wolff, R. J., 19
World Health Organization
 (WHO), 9, 26
Worner, T. M., 85

Yablonsky, L., 60
Yang, M. M. P., 43, 83

Zinberg, N. E., 55, 79, 80
Zucker, D. K., 73